LEARN HAND-READING
THE EASY WAY
PALMISTRY IN PICTURES

**Other Books by the author
in UBSPD**

Dial Your Birth Number

Encyclopaedia of Palm and Palm Reading

Numerology, Palmistry and Prosperity

Palmistry, Marriage and Family Welfare

LEARN HAND READING THE EASY WAY
PALMISTRY IN PICTURES

M. Katakkar

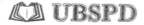

UBS Publishers' Distributors Ltd.
New Delhi • Bangalore • Chennai • Calcutta •
Patna • Kanpur • London

UBS Publishers' Distributors Ltd.
5 Ansari Road, New Delhi-110 002
Phones: 3273601, 3266646 ☆ *Cable*: ALLBOOKS ☆
Fax: 3276593, 3274261
e-mail: ubspd.del@del3.vsnl.net.in ☆ Internet: www.ubspd.com
10 First Main Road, Gandhi Nagar, Bangalore-560 009
Phones: 2263901, 2263902, 2253903 ☆ *Cable*: ALLBOOKS ☆
Fax: 2263904
6, Sivaganga Road, Nungambakkam, Chennai-600 034
Phones : 8276355, 8270189 ☆ *Cable* : UBSIPUB ☆ *Fax* : 8278920
8/1-B, Chowringhee Lane, Calcutta-700 016
Phones: 2441821, 2442910, 2449473 ☆ *Cable*: UBSIPUBS ☆
Fax : 2450027 ☆ e-mail: ubspdcal @ cal. vsnl.net.in
5 A, Rajendra Nagar, Patna-800 016
Phones: 672856, 673973, 656170 ☆ *Cable* : UBSPUB ☆ *Fax*: 656169
80, Noronha Road, Cantonment, Kanpur-208 004
Phones : 369124, 362665, 357588 ☆ *Fax* : 315122

Distributors for Western India:
M/s Preface Books
Shivali Apartments, Plot No. 1, S. No. 25/4, Chintamani Society,
Karve Nagar, Pune-411052

Overseas Contact
475 North Circular Road, Neasden, London NW2 7QG
Tele : 081-450-8667 ☆ *Fax* : 0181-452-6612 Attn: UBS

© Dr. M. Katakkar

1999 Edition

M. Katakkar asserts the moral right to be
identified as the author of this work

All rights reserved. No part of this publication may be reproduced or
transmitted in any form or by any means, electronic or mechanical
including photocopying, recording, or any information storage and
retrieval system, without permission in writing from the publisher.

Cover Design : UBS Art Studio

Designed & Typeset at UBSPD in 12 pt. Goudy
Printed at Nutech Photolithographers Delhi (India)

CONTENTS

Introduction	
General Map of the Hand	Fig. 1
Lines on the Hand	Fig. 2
Star and Cross on the Hand	Fig. 3
Shape of the Hand	Figs. 4-11
Divisions of the Hand	Figs. 12-14
The Fingers	Figs. 15-21
The Thumb	Figs. 22-30
Square Hand with Different Fingers	Figs. 31-37
Spacing between the Fingers	Figs. 38-46
Loops on Fingers	Figs. 47-51
Mounts on the Hand	Figs. 52-58
Rings of Solomon and Saturn	Figs. 59-60
Flat Zone of Thought	Fig. 61
Lines and Stars on Fingers	Figs. 62-76
The Quadrangle	Figs. 77-78
The Big Triangle and the Signs in the Triangle	Figs. 79-94
Defects in the Line	Fig. 95
Good Signs on the Hand	Fig. 96
Zodical Signs and Months on Fingers	Fig. 97
Time Factor on Hand	Fig. 98
The Line of Life	Figs. 99-167
Lines of Influence	Figs. 168-186
The Line of Head	Figs. 187-260
The Line of Fate	Figs. 261-305
The Line of Heart	Figs. 306-349
The Line of Sun	Figs. 350-371
The Line of Mercury	Figs. 372-397
The Line of Mars	Figs. 398-404

Via Lasciva	Fig. 405
Girdle of Venus	Figs. 406-409
The Line of Intuition	Figs. 410-411
The Bracelet	Fig. 412
The Lines of Travel	Figs. 413-416
Miscellaneous Signs	Figs. 417-418
The Line of Marriage	Figs. 419-427
The Lines of Children	Fig. 428

INDEX OF SIGNS ON THE HAND

ALPHABETICAL INDEX

INTRODUCTION

There are several books on the subject of hand-reading but the study of these books involves strenuous study, patience and considerable time. Sometimes the study also requires an instructor to coach. Such a laborious procedure may sometimes lead to boredom, frustration and finally leaving the subject half-learned.

It was therefore my desire to produce such a work on palmistry that could make it very easy to learn the subject and which could be studied during one's leisure time. The motive was to make the subject more interesting and at the same time more simple and instructive.

This book therefore is a novel idea. The pictures given here are sufficient for the knowledge of the subject, which is based on both the Indian and the Western systems of palmistry.

The Index of Signs on the Hand and the Alphabetical Index, both at the end of the book, will prove very useful.

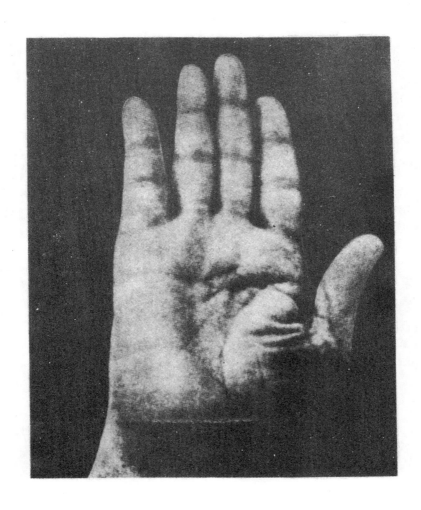

THE HAND OF MAHATMA GANDHI
The Father of the Nation

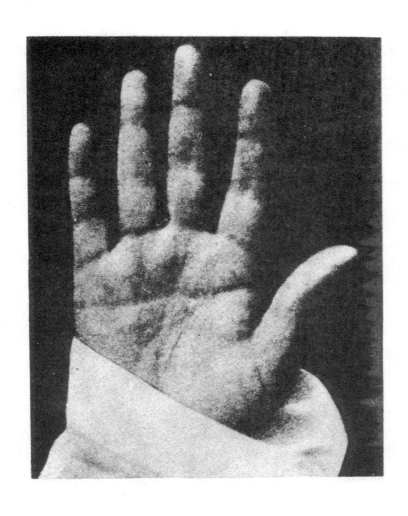

THE HAND OF SHAIKH MUJIBUR REHMAN
The First President of Bangladesh

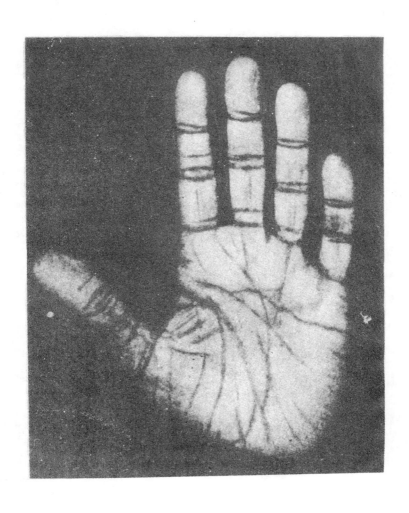

THE HAND OF DR. S. RADHAKRISHNAN
The Ex-President of India

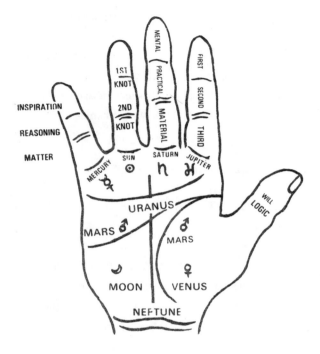

Fig. 1
General Map of the Hand
Mounts and their signs

Fig. 2: THE LINES ON THE HAND

There are six main lines on the hand

1. The Line of Heart: It deals with emotions, sentiments and feelings
2. The Line of Head: It deals with logic, reason, and practical thinking
3. The Line of Life: It deals with health and longevity
4. The Line of Fate: It deals with career and prosperity
5. The Line of Sun: It deals with success, art, and literary career
6. The Line of Mercury: It deals with business, intelligence and health

There are seven minor lines on the hand

1. The Line of Mars: This line is inside the Line of Life and shows good health
2. Via Lasciva: It deals with the lower instincts
3. The Girdle of Venus: It deals with emotions and sexual feelings
4. The Line of Travel: It indicates journey or travel
5. The Line of Intuition: It shows gift of inner-voice
6. The Line of Marriage: It deals with married life
7. The Lines of Children: They tell about children

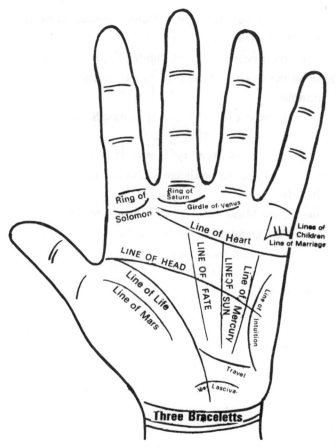

**Fig. 2
Lines on the Hand**

FIG. 3: STAR AND CROSS ON THE HAND

1. Star on the Mount of Jupiter: Public honour, fame and wealthy marriage
2. Star on the first phalange of Jupiter finger: Travels
3. Star on the negative Mount of Mars: Military honours
4. Star at the base of the Mount of Venus: Success in love
5. Star on the line of Mercury: Unexpected luck
6. Cross on the second phalange of Jupiter finger: Rich friends
7. Cross on the Mount of Jupiter: Happy marriage
8. Cross in the Quadrangle under the Mount of Saturn:
   (a) Fortunate and lucky life
   (b) Priesthood
   (c) Occultism

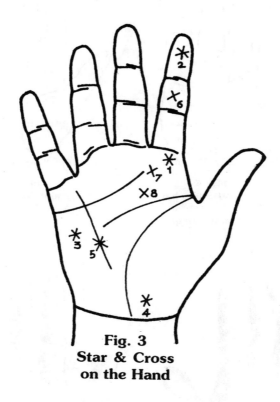

**Fig. 3
Star & Cross
on the Hand**

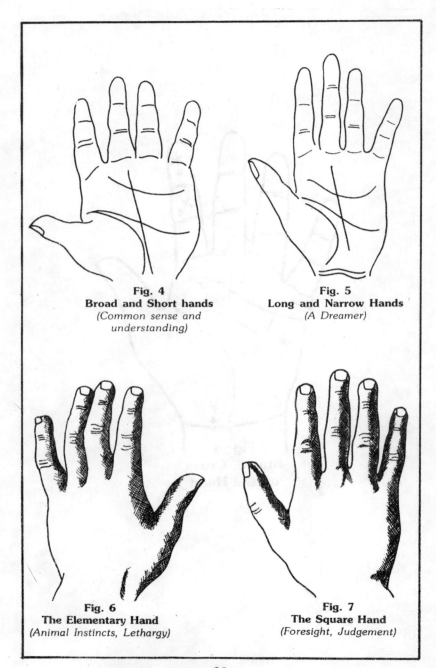

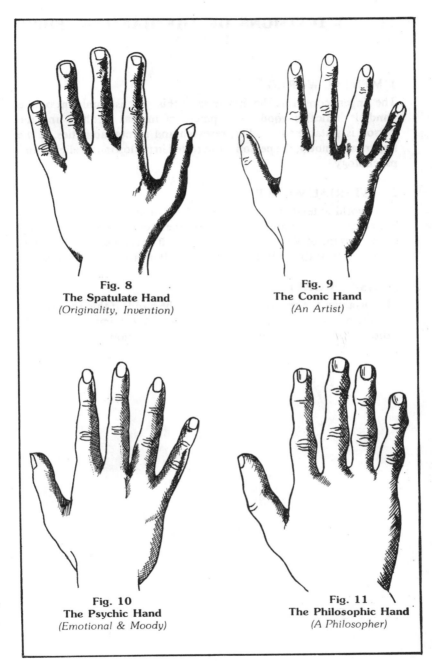

Fig. 8
The Spatulate Hand
(Originality, Invention)

Fig. 9
The Conic Hand
(An Artist)

Fig. 10
The Psychic Hand
(Emotional & Moody)

Fig. 11
The Philosophic Hand
(A Philosopher)

FIG. 12: DIVISIONS OF THE HAND — FIRST SYSTEM

1 MENTAL WORLD
The fingers constitute the first zone. If this zone is dominant on the hand, it indicates good development of mental faculties and the person is suitable for studies, research and mental activities. If the fingers are knotty, the person is interested in philosophy, religion and psychology.

2 MATERIAL WORLD
This world extends from the base of the fingers to the imaginary horizontal line running from the top of the Mount of Moon to the top of the Mount of Venus. If this zone is well developed, the person is more practical than idealistic and runs after fame and money.

3 BASAL WORLD
This occupies the remaining portion of the hand. If this zone is very prominent, it shows poor intellect and little common-sense. It indicates a person who is vulgar in talk and action.

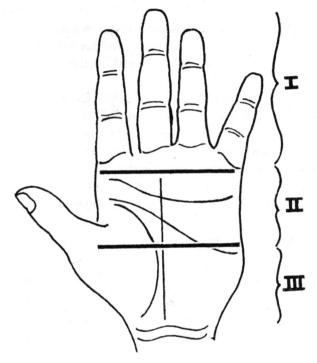

**Fig. 12
Division of the Hand — First System**

FIG. 13: DIVISIONS OF THE HAND — SECOND SYSTEM

1 **Conscious Zone:** This zone comprises the Mounts of Jupiter, the positive Mount of Mars, the Mount of Venus, the finger of Jupiter and the thumb. Jupiter shows ambition, religion, honour, prestige. Mars shows courage, dash, activity, enthusiasm and a hot-tempered nature. The Mount of Venus indicates passion, sex, sympathy, love for beauty, art and culture. The greater or less development of these Mounts increases or decreases the above characteristics.

2 **Social Zone:** The Fate Line travels through this zone. The development of this zone and a good Fate Line shows social temperament. This zone comprises the Mount of Neptune, the Mount of Uranus and the Mount of Saturn. They indicate religion, mysticism and common-sense respectively.

3 **Sub-conscious Zone:** This zone comprises the Mount of Mercury, half of the Mount of Apollo, the negative Mount of Mars and the Mount of Moon. Apollo shows intelligence, creativity, literary activity, oratory. Mercury indicates business talents, shrewdness and intuition. Negative Mars indicates defence, nervousness and patience. Moon presents coolness, imagination and moodiness.

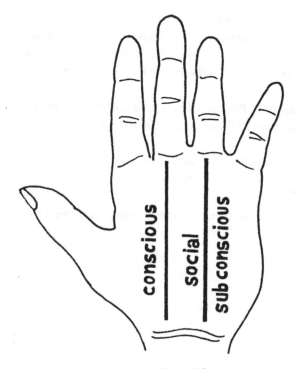

**Fig. 13
Division of the Hand — Second System**

FIG. 14: DIVISIONS OF THE HAND – THIRD SYSTEM

1 Zone of Thought: Development of this zone indicates a promising career. Flat zone shows no ambition (Fig. 61).

2 Zone of Action: It lies between the lines of Heart and Head. A balanced zone indicates a desire for higher aspects and endows higher ideals in life. Triangle attached to the Heart line in this zone means income. Falling lines from the Heart line mean lack of judgement.

3 Zone of Impulse: Parallel lines to Life line mean happiness, many brothers, sisters and friends. Cross lines show difficulties.

4 Zone of Imagination: It signifies a love for the beautiful, high ideals, a love for travel and change.

5 Zone of the Thumb: It deals with ego, will-power, reason and logic.

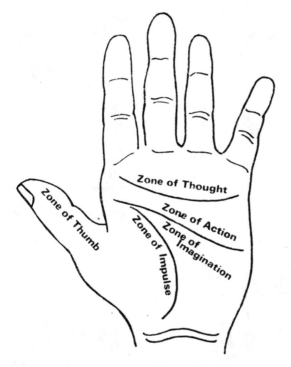

**Fig. 14
Division of the Hand — Third System**

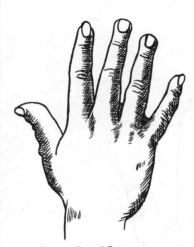

**Fig. 15
The Mixed Hand**
(Jack of all trades)

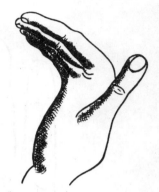

**Fig. 16
Flexible Fingers**
(Adaptability)

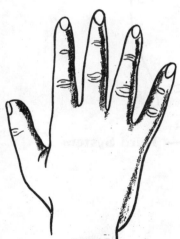

**Fig. 17
Smooth Fingers**
(Inspiration)

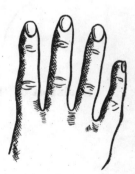

**Fig. 18
Knotty Fingers**
(Maturity of Thought)

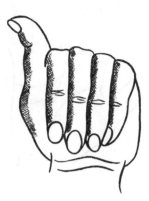

**Fig. 19
Long Fingers**
(Slow & sensitive)

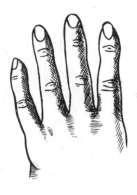

**Fig. 20
Fingers with first knot developed**
(Systematic and Careful Thinking)

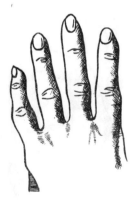

**Fig. 21
Fingers with second knot developed**
(Method and order in work)

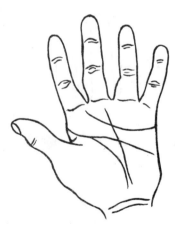

**Fig. 22
High Set Thumb**
(Mean minded and selfish)

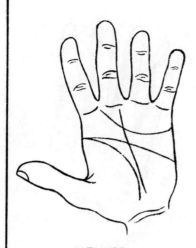

**Fig. 23
Low Set Thumb**
(Sympathy and generosity)

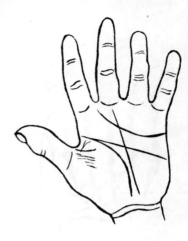

**Fig. 24
Medium Set Thumb**
(Balanced Mind)

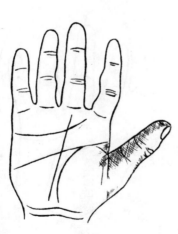

**Fig. 25
Strongly developed Thumb**
(Willpower and confidence)

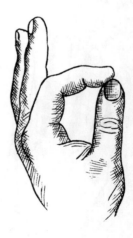

**Fig. 26
The diplomatic Thumb**
(Tact and diplomacy)

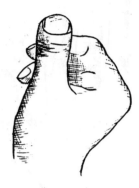

Fig. 27
The clubbed Thumb
(Cruelty)

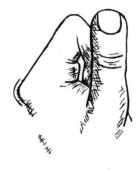

Fig. 28
Paddle shaped Thumb
(Determination and tenacity)

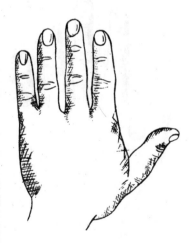

Fig. 29
The nervous Thumb
(Lack of confidence)

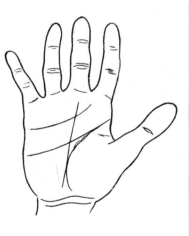

Fig. 30
The Waistlike Thumb
(Talents and good manners)

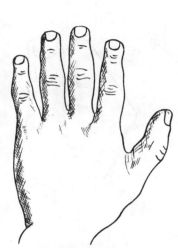

Fig. 31
The Square hand with
short-square fingers
(Quick grasp but scrupulous)

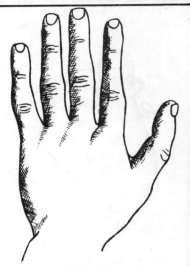

Fig. 32
The Square hand with long
square fingers
(Good logic and reasoning)

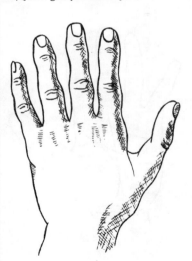

Fig. 33
The Square hand with
knotty fingers
(Analytic Mind)

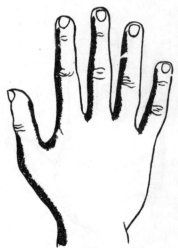

Fig. 34
The Square hand with
spatulate fingers
(Invention and originality)

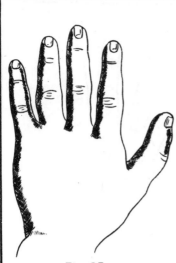

Fig. 35
The square hand with conic fingers
(Method in art and poetry)

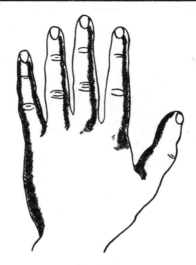

Fig. 36
The square hand with Psychic fingers
(Clash between idealism and materialism)

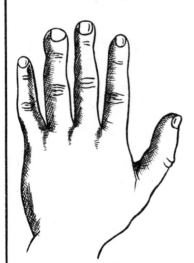

Fig. 37
The square hand with mixed fingers
(Versatility)

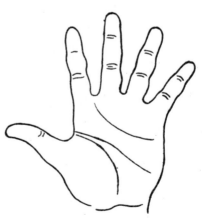

Fig. 38
Wide space between thumb & Jupiter finger
(Sympathy & generosity)

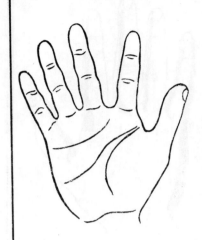

**Fig. 39
Wide space between Jupiter
& Saturn fingers**
(Man of thought)

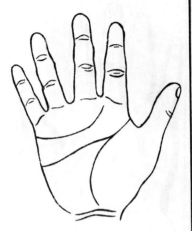

**Fig. 40
Wide space between Saturn
& Apollo fingers**
(Carelessness about future)

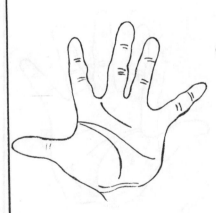

**Fig. 41
Wide space between Apollo
& Mercury fingers**
(Man of action)

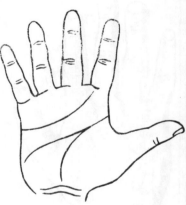

**Fig. 42
Equal spacing between
fingers**
(Balanced nature)

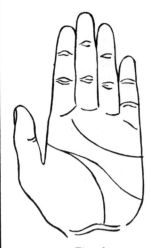

Fig. 43
Fingers closed together
(Stiff and selfish attitude)

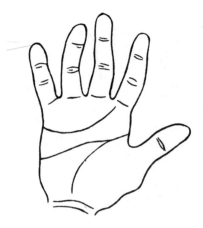

Fig. 44
Saturn and Apollo fingers leaning towards each other
(Secretive disposition)

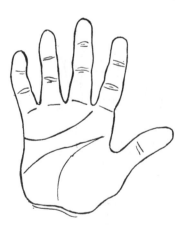

Fig. 45
Mercury finger leaning towards Apollo finger
(Talent in business)

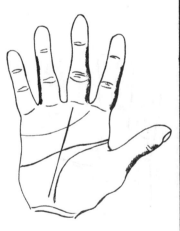

Fig. 46
Twisted fingers
(Critical nature)

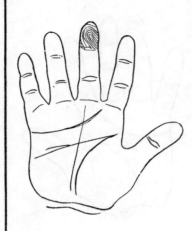

**Fig. 47
Loops on fingers**
(Nervous troubles)

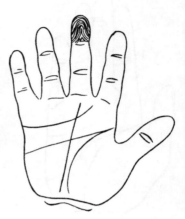

**Fig. 48
Tented arch on fingers**
(Nervousness)

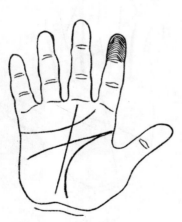

**Fig. 49
Arch type formation of
Papillary ridges**
(Faulty blood circulation)

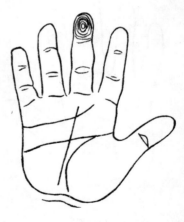

**Fig. 50
Whorls on fingers**
(Heart troubles)

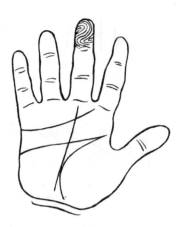

Fig. 51
Composite type formation
of Papillary ridges
(A Glutton)

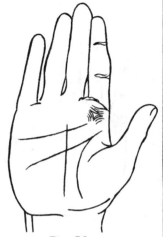

Fig. 52
The Mount of Jupiter
(Ambition, dignity, honour, prestige, religion)

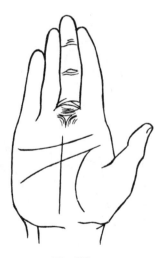

Fig. 53
The Mount of Saturn
(Philosophy, Melancholiness, Soberness, Balanced mind)

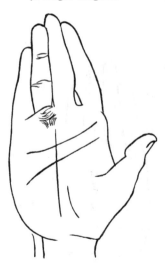

Fig. 54
The Mount of Apollo
(Art, Success, Originality, Oratory)

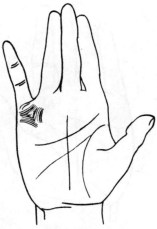

Fig. 55
The Mount of Mercury
(Shrewdness, Cunningness, Business ability, Love of Science)

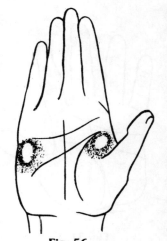

Fig. 56
The Mounts of Mars
(Dash, courage, energy, activity, hot temper, erratic)

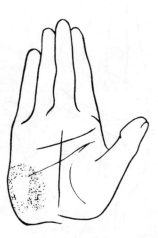

Fig. 57
The Mount of Moon
(Imagination, moodiness, Love of travel, a dreamer)

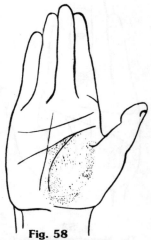

Fig. 58
The Mount of Venus
(Love, art, beauty, compassion, sex)

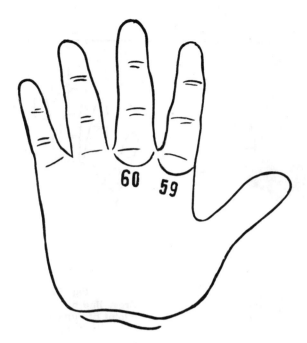

Fig. 59
Ring of Solomon

Fig. 60
Ring of Saturn

FIGS. 59 AND 60

Fig. 59: The ring of Solomon indicates deep interest in occult sciences, psychic powers. It also shows wisdom, knowledge and generosity.

Fig. 60: The ring of Saturn shows troubles and unhappiness in one's career and suicidal tendencies. It reduces the qualities of the Mount of Saturn which are sobriety, wisdom and a balanced mind.

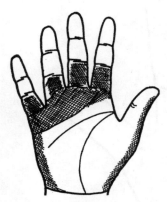

Fig. 61
Flat zone of thought
(No ambition)

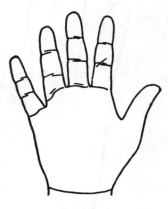

Fig. 62
Cross line on the second joint of Jupiter finger
(Harmful & dishonest attitude)

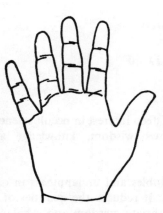

Fig. 63
Cross line on the third joint of Jupiter finger
(Acquisition of other's money)

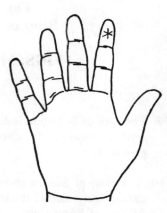

Fig. 64
A star on the first phalange of Jupiter finger
(Wide travel, fame & honour)

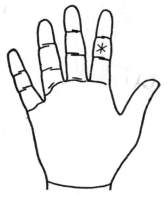

Fig. 65
A star on the second
phalange of Jupiter finger
(Good luck & wealth)

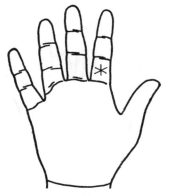

Fig. 66
A star on the third phalange
of Jupiter finger
(Immorality)

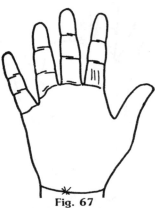

Fig. 67
Three vertical lines on the
third phalange of Jupiter
finger and a star on the
Rascette
(Acquisition of other's money)

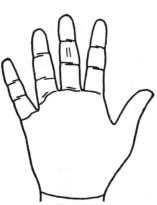

Fig. 68
Two vertical lines on the
second phalange of Saturn
finger
(Success in difficult enterprise)

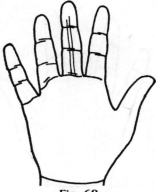

Fig. 69
Few lines from root to the first phalange of Saturn finger
(Success in mineral business)

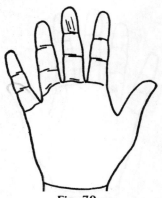

Fig. 70
Vertical lines on first phalange of Saturn finger
(Jealousy)

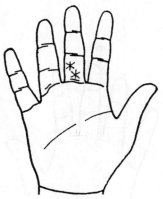

Fig. 71
Two stars on the third phalange of Saturn finger with a break in Head line under Saturn Mount
a) On woman's hand:- Suicide in water
b) On man's hand:- Death

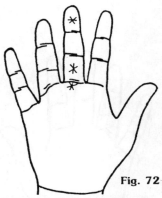

Fig. 72
A star on first phalange of Saturn finger
A star on third phalange of Saturn finger
A star at the root of Saturn finger
a) Unhappiness
b) Death through weapon
c) Sterility of the wife

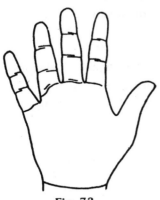

Fig. 73
Spot on Saturn finger
(Theft by one in the family)

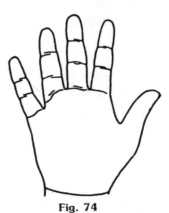

Fig. 74
Island on the II joint of Saturn finger
(Wealth through adoption or lottery)

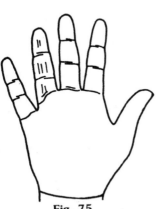

Fig. 75
Lines on the finger of Apollo
(Wealth, fame & luck)

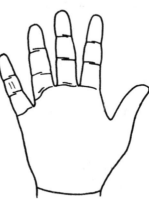

Fig. 76
Two or three vertical lines on the second phalange of Mercury finger
(Pursuit in occult subject)

FIG. 77: THE QUADRANGLE

Position on the Hand: It occupies the space between the lines of Heart and Head. This is the same zone of Action shown in Fig. 14.

2 (a) Narrow Quadrangle: This is found on the hands of religious persons. It also indicates prejudice. injustice and bigotry.
A narrow Quadrangle with a poor line of Mercury indicates asthma.

(b) Broad Quadrangle: This is a sign of broadmindedness.

(c) Very Broad Quadrangle: This shows carelessness in ideas and thoughts.

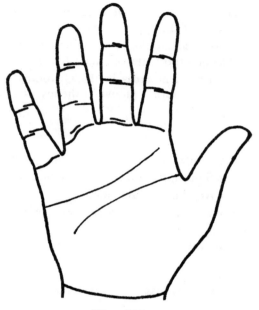

**Fig. 77
The Quadrangle**

FIG. 78: THE SIGNS IN THE QUADRANGLE

1 Cross:

   (a) A cross in the Quadrangle touching the line of Heart signifies influence of the opposite sex.
   (b) A cross touching the Fate line under the Mount of Saturn speaks of a fortunate and lucky life and a religious attitude.
   (c) An independent cross in the Quadrangle and under the Mount of Saturn is known as the mystic cross. It gives love for occultism.

2 Star:
   (a) Under Jupiter, it promises pride and power.
   (b) Under Saturn, it promises wordly success.
   (c) Under Apollo, it means fame.
   (d) Under Mercury, it indicates success in scientific pursuits.

3 Square: It indicates sympathetic nature and quick grasp of things.

4 Triangle: It shows love for deep studies.

5 Circle: It means eye trouble. Three circles touching each other mean epilepsy.

6 Grill: It presages madness.

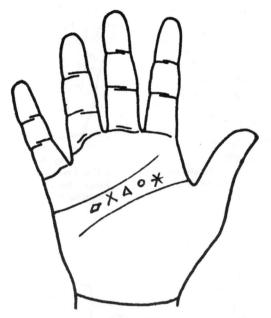

**Fig. 78
Signs in the Quadrangle**

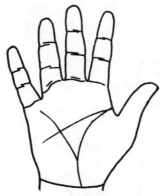

Fig. 79
The Big Triangle consists of Lines of Life, Head & Mercury

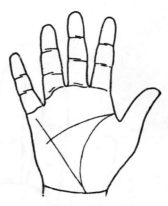

Fig. 80
The Big Triangle occupying larger space on hand
(Good luck and long life)

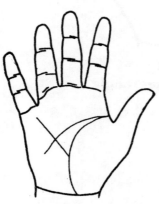

Fig. 81
The Big Triangle occupying smaller space on hand
(Timidity, cowardice)

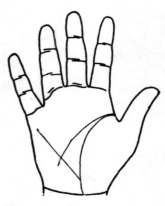

Fig. 82
The Big Triangle at a very low position on hand
(Lethargy)

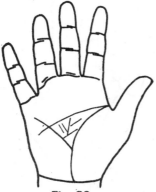

Fig. 83
Many lines in the Big Triangle
(Sensitivity, impatience, fretfulness)

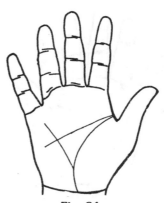

Fig. 84
Wide angle between Life & Head lines
(Dull intellect & blunt nature)

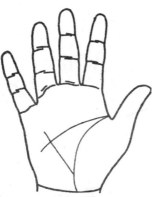

Fig. 85
Well defined angle between Head and Mercury lines
(Vivacity, good health)

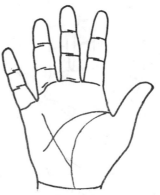

Fig. 86
Obtuse angle between Head & Mercury lines
(Ultranervous disposition)

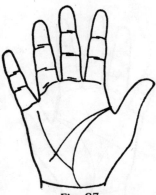

Fig. 87
Head & Mercury lines form an angle on the Mount of Moon
(Catarrh, epilepsy, mental, paralysis)

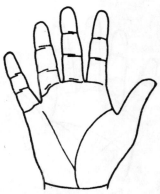

Fig. 88
Life and Mercury lines forming a narrow angle
(Ill health, feeble mindedness)

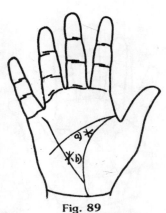

Fig. 89
a) A star in the Big Triangle
b) A star in the Big Triangle touching Mercury line.
a) Riches   b) Blindness

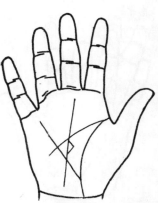

Fig. 90
A triangle in the Big Triangle and between the lines of Fate & Life
(Military Renown)

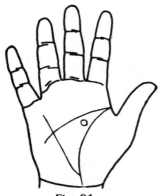

Fig. 91
Circle in the Big Triangle
(Troubles from opposite sex)

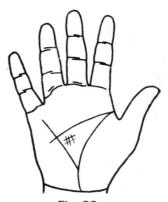

Fig. 92
Grill in the Big Triangle
(Hidden enemies)

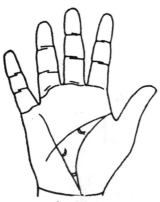

Fig. 93
A Crescent in the Big Triangle
a) **Touching Mercury line**
(Good luck & success)
b) **Touching Head line**
(Violent death)
c) **In the lower angle**
(Infidelity)

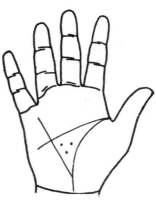

Fig. 94
Red dots in the Big Triangle
(Pregnancy)

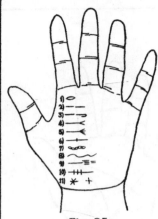

Fig. 95
Defects in the line:-
1) Island 2) Break
3) Broken end turning back
4) Fork 5) Tassel 6) Dot
7) Chained line 8) Wavy line
9) Capillary lines 10) Cross bars 11) Star & Cross

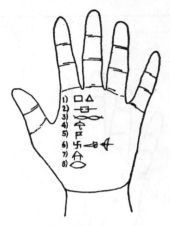

Fig. 96
Good signs on the Hand
1) Square & Triangle 2) A break protected by square
3) Two Fish 4) Umbrella
5) Flag 6) Swastik — Sword — Bow & 7) Temple 8) Yava

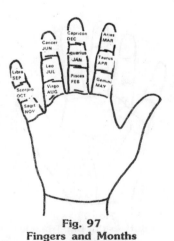

Fig. 97
Fingers and Months
Fingers and Zodical signs

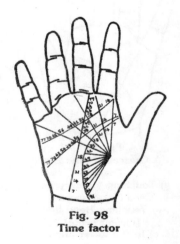

Fig. 98
Time factor

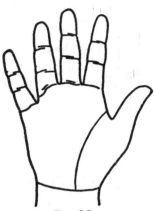

**Fig. 99
Straight line of Life**
(Cold nature)

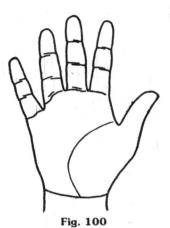

**Fig. 100
Life line covering greater portion of the Mount of Venus**
(Excess vitality and greater sex urge)

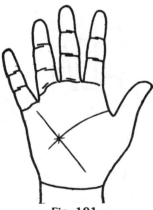

**Fig. 101
Star at the Intersection of Head line and the Mercury line**
(Childlessness)

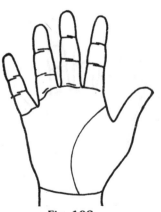

**Fig. 102
Life line starting high on the Jupiter Mount**
(Ambition, dictatorship & cruelty)

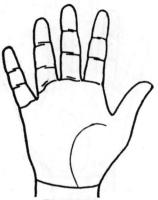

Fig. 103
Life line starting from the Mount of Mars
(Struggle & hardship, poor health)

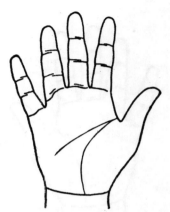

Fig. 104
Life line and Head line connected at the start
(Good logic & reasoning, caution, prudence)

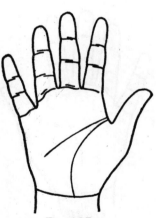

Fig. 105
Small space between Head and Life lines.
(Dash and independent nature)

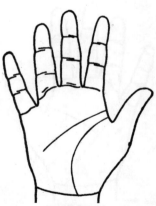

Fig. 106
Wide gap between Head & Life line
(Vanity, hasty & quarrelsome nature)

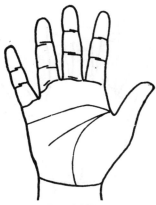

Fig. 107
Joining of Life, Head and Heart lines
(Nervous & sincere nature, also sudden death)

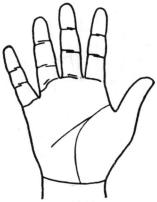

Fig. 108
Life & Head lines run together
(Sensitivity, diffident & timidity)

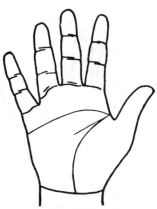

Fig. 109
Life line joined to the Heart line with short Head line
(Sickness or accident)

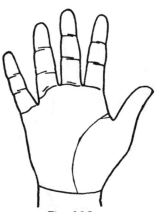

Fig. 110
Fork at the start of the Life line
(Fidelity & justice)

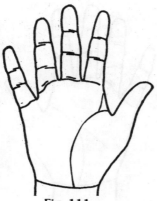

Fig. 111
Life line starting with
a deepfork on Jupiter
(Successful life)

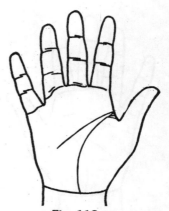

Fig. 112
Two or more forks at the
beginning, below line of
Head
(Honour to the parents)

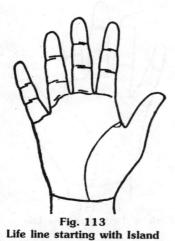

Fig. 113
Life line starting with Island
(Mystery of birth)

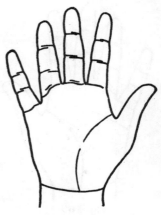

Fig. 114
Break in the Life line
*(Change in life due to accident
or sickness or travel)*

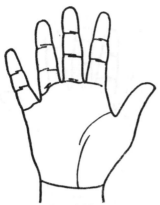

Fig. 115
Overlapping the break
(Overcoming the danger)

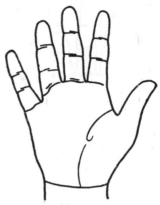

Fig. 116
Break with a hook in the Life line
(Fatal accident)

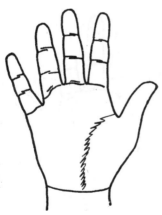

Fig. 117
Ladder like formation in the Life line
(Ill health)

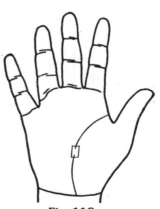

Fig. 118
Square on a break
(Protection from danger)

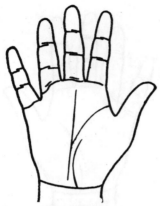

Fig. 119
Broken end of Life line joining the Fate line
(Danger avoided by good luck)

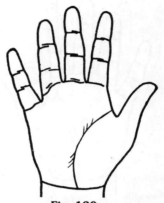

Fig. 120
Rising & Falling lines
(Change for better or worse)

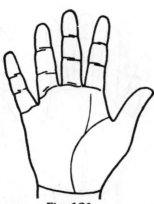

Fig. 121
Rising branch from Life line going to the Jupiter Mount
(Success & realisation of ambition)

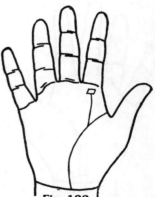

Fig. 122
Rising branch from Life line going to clear square on Jupiter
(Lucid expression of a good teacher)

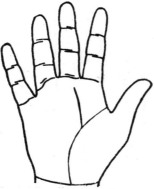

Fig. 123
Rising branch from Life line going to the Mount of Saturn
(Marital success & monetary stability)

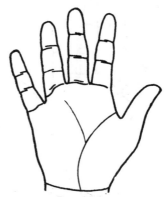

Fig. 124
Rising branch from Life line going to the Mount of Sun
(Success, glory & wealth)

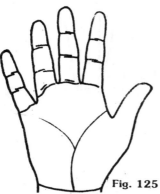

Fig. 125
Rising branch from Life line going to the Mount of Mercury
(Success in business or in scientific pursuits)

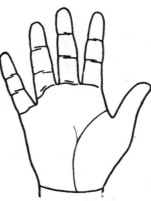

Fig. 126
Rising branch from Life line going to the Mount of Uranus
(Success in life)

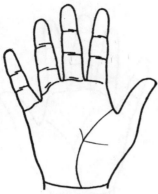

Fig. 127
Rising branch from
Life line connected by a line
from Venus joining each
other on Life line
(Family attachment)

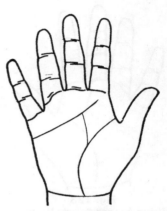

Fig. 128
Rising branch stopped by
Heart line
(Misjudgement in affection)

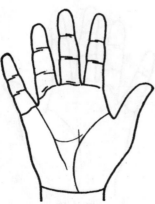

Fig. 129
Rising branch cut by a
line from Mercury line
(Loss of enterprise)

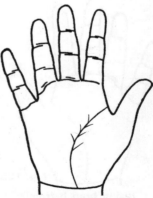

Fig. 130
Rising lines from both sides
of the Life line
(Riches & good health)

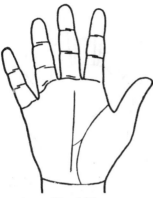

Fig. 131
Falling sprout from Life
line, joining the Fate line
(Regaining health)

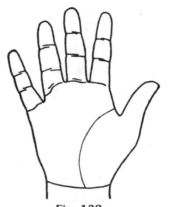

Fig. 132
A line from Jupiter
touching the Life line
(Lung & chest trouble)

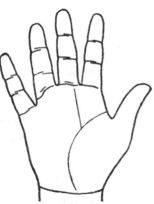

Fig. 133
A Line from Saturn
touching the Life line
(Tooth trouble)

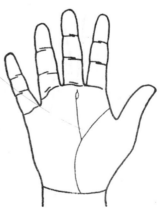

Fig. 134
Island on Saturn on the
line joining the Life line
(Danger from animals)

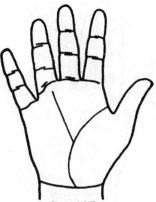

Fig. 135
Line from Sun touching
the Life Line
(Eye trouble)

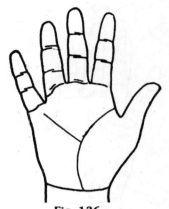

Fig. 136
Line from Mercury touching
the Life line
(Bilious & nerve troubles)

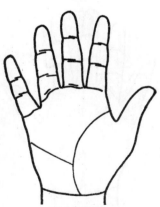

Fig. 137
Line from Negative Mount
of Mars touching the Life
line
(Wound)

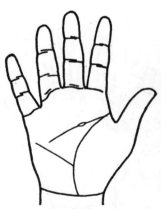

Fig. 138
Line from Negative Mount
of Mars with island on Head
line
(Wound to the head)

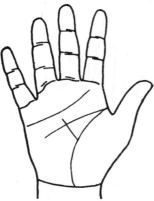

Fig. 139
Line from plain of Mars
touching the Life line
(Accident)

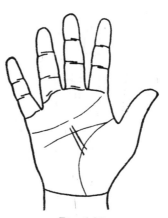

Fig. 140
Two parallel lines from
Uranus cutting the Life line
*(Strange & unexpected
favourable happenings)*

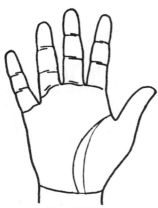

Fig. 141
Branch from the beginning
of the Life line upto
Bracellet
(Severe headaches)

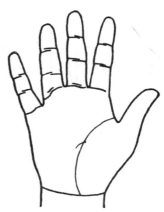

Fig. 142
Falling branch from a black
spot on Life line
(Chronic complaints)

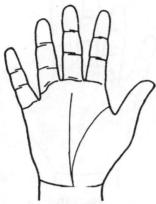

Fig. 143
Fate line touching Life line on the Mount of Neptune
(Success & fortune)

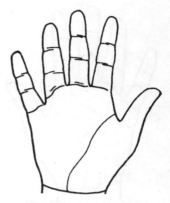

Fig. 144
Life line taking a turn on Mount of Moon & reaching rascettes
(Love for travel)

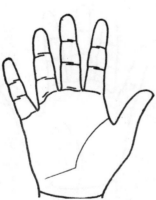

Fig. 145
Life line suddenly going at right angles on the Mount of Moon
(Epilepsy)

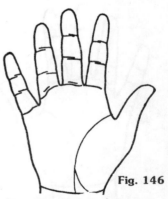

Fig. 146
Neptunian Life line Forked one prong to Mount of Venus
(Clash between married partners)

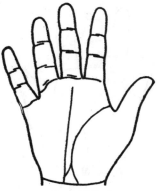

Fig. 147
One fork of the line of Life merging into Fate line
(Dull ending of life)

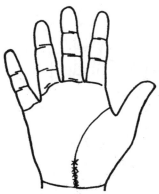

Fig. 148
Life line ending in series of crosses
(Poverty in old age)

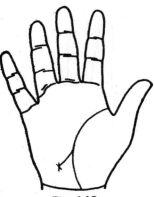

Fig. 149
Cross at the end of the line coming out from Life line
(Sudden death)

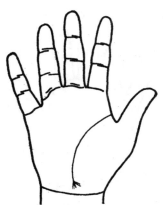

Fig. 150
Life line ending in Tassel
(Violent death or murder or execution)

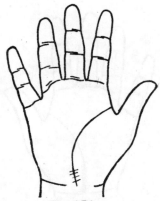

Fig. 151
Life line ending in cross bar
(Sudden or unexpected death)

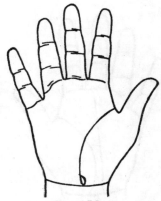

Fig. 152
Life line ending in an Island
(Hysteria)

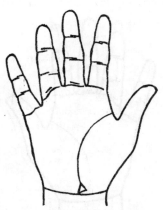

Fig. 153
Triangle at the end of Life line
(Falsehood)

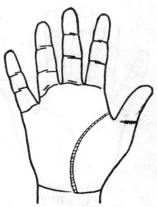

Fig. 154
A broad & shallow Life line
(Lack of resistance to disease)

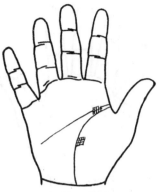

Fig. 155
Grills on Head line & Venus Mount both touching life line
(Change of religion)

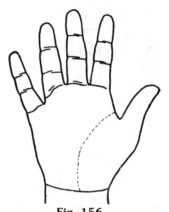

Fig. 156
Life line formed by small lines
(Intense nervousness)

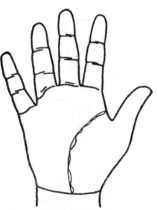

Fig. 157
Chained line of Life
(Disturbing health)

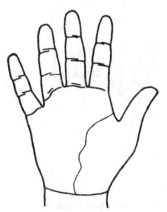

Fig. 158
Wavy line of Life
(Ups & downs in health)

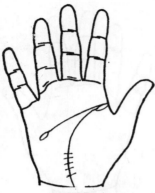

Fig. 159
Island at the beginning of Life line & also at the end of Head line with many bars in the Life line
(Deafness & Dumbness)

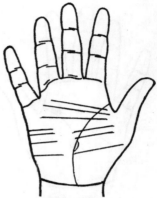

Fig. 160
Island on Life line & hand full of cross lines
(Nervousness)

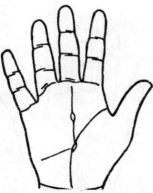

Fig. 161
Islanded line from Saturn Joins on Island on the Life line & another line from middle Moon joins the island
(Gout & Rheumatism)

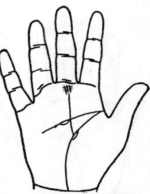

Fig. 162
A line from a grill on the Mount of Saturn joining an Island on the Life line with dots or Island on the Head line
(Paralysis)

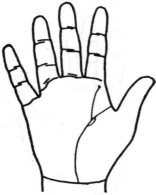

Fig. 163
A line joining a red dot on Jupiter & an island on Life line
(Apoplexy)

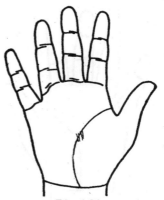

Fig. 164
Hedge Formation on Life line
(Asthma)

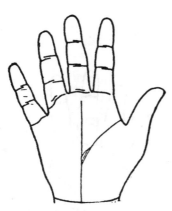

Fig. 165
Short Life line ending abruptly by capillary lines & these capillary lines joined to Fate line starting from Rascettes
(Danger to life avoided by good luck)

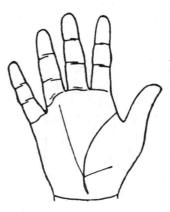

Fig. 166
A line from Mount of Venus meeting the Sun line on the Life line
(Popularity and reputation to wife)

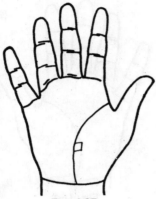

Fig. 167
A square touching Life line from inside
(Imprisonment)

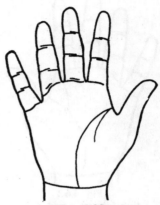

Fig. 168
A Vertical line of Influence from beginning of Life line
(Influence of parents)

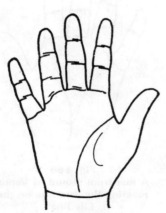

Fig. 169
A Vertical line of Influence turning away from Life line
(Withdrawal of influence)

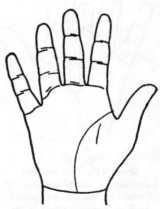

Fig. 170
A Vertical line of Influence on Positive Mount of Mars
(Influence of a male)

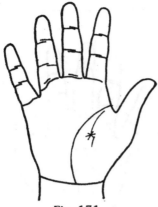

Fig. 171
If an Influence line rising early on Positive Mars ends in a star, & has another line by its side, but away from Life line which grows shorter after the star
(Death of father or mother)

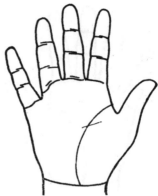

Fig. 172
Cross line on the Mount of Mars cutting the Life line
(Blood pressure)

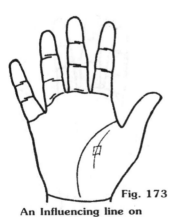

Fig. 173
An Influencing line on Mount of Venus entering a square & coming out of it from other end
(Imprisonment to influencing person)

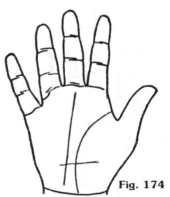

Fig. 174
Horizontal line from Venus Mount cuts line of Life & the Fate line
(Loss due to influencing person)

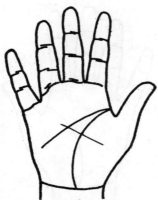

Fig. 175
Horizontal line from Venus cutting the line of Head
(Interference in plans)

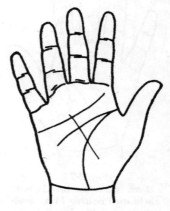

Fig. 176
Horizontal line from Venus cutting the Heart line
(Interference in love)

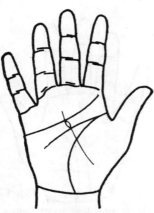

Fig. 177
Island in the horizontal line cutting Heart line
(Disgraceful liaison)

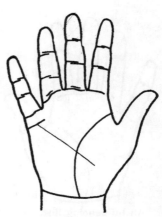

Fig. 178
Horizontal cross line from Venus touching the Marriage line
(Unhappy married life)

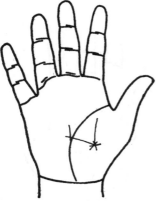

Fig. 179
Cross line from Venus
starting from a star at the
end of Influence line &
cutting a rising branch on
Life line
(Death of a relative obstructs career)

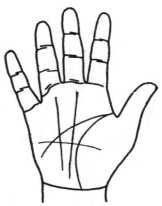

Fig. 180
Cross line from Venus
cutting the lines of Fate
Head, Sun & ending on
upper Mount of Mars
(Wound due to relative or friend)

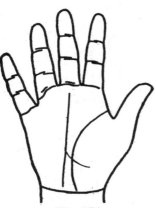

Fig. 181
A line from Venus Mount
crossing the Life line and
merging in Fate line
(Interference in career)

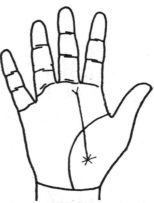

Fig. 182
Cross line starting from a
star on Mount of Venus and
ending in Fork on the
Mount of Saturn
(Death or insanity of the partner)

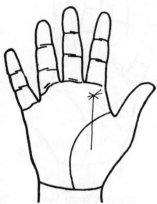

Fig. 183
Cross line ending in a star on the Mount of Jupiter
(Ambition crowned with success)

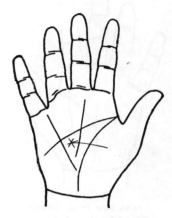

Fig. 184
Cross line ending on a star in the Triangle but after crossing the line of Fate
(Loss of money)

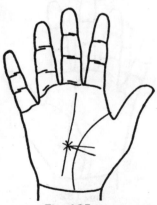

Fig. 185
Two lines from Mount of Venus which meet in a star on the line of Fate
(Two love affairs met with frustration)

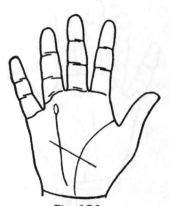

Fig. 186
Cross line from Venus Mount cutting Sun line ending in island
(Scandal due to guilty intrigue)

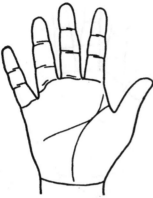

Fig. 187
Head line from Jupiter but touching the Life line
(Powerful mind)

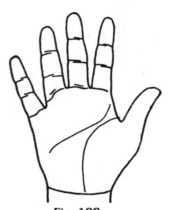

Fig. 188
Head line from Jupiter but slightly separated from Line of Life
(Impetuous & hasty nature)

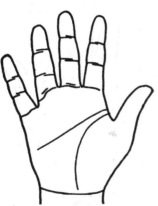

Fig. 189
Wide distance between Life and Head
(Foolhardiness & overconfidence)

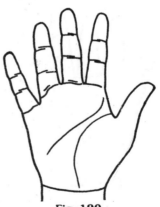

Fig. 190
Head line from Jupiter away from Life line and sloping to the Mount of Moon
(Obstinacy & quarrelsome disposition)

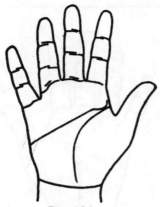

Fig. 191
Head line with a curve
under the Mount of Jupiter
and going right across the
hand without touching the
Life line
(Extravagance & conceit)

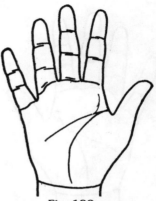

Fig. 192
Line from Jupiter joining
the Head line
(Desire to become great)

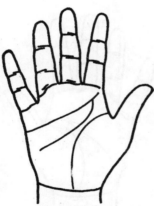

Fig. 193
Head line from Jupiter
touching the Heart line on
Jupiter
(Harmony in love & duty)

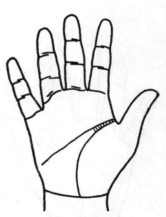

Fig. 194
Head line, not touching
the line of Life but is
connected by minor
lines or branches
(Evil temper)

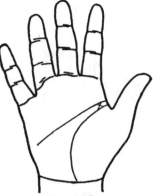

Fig. 195
Cross joining the Head line
and the Life line
(Serious family troubles)

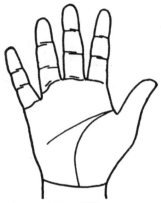

Fig. 196
Head line closely connected
to Life line
(Sensitive nature)

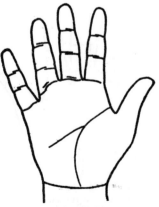

Fig. 197
Head line starting from Life
line
(Neglected education)

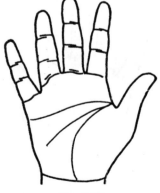

Fig. 198
Life line, Head line and
Heart line connected to
each other at the start
(Sudden death)

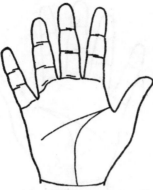

Fig. 199
Head line closely connected to Life line and running together for sometime
(Family dominance)

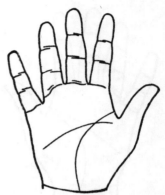

Fig. 200
Head line starting from inside the Life line or from the Mount of Mars
(Timidity & shyness)

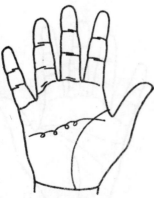

Fig. 201
Head line starting from inside the line of Life and across the hand in a winding and wavy way.
(Violent resolutions)

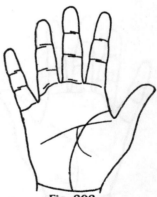

Fig. 202
A Head line which starts from inside Life line having a branch which goes to the Mount of Venus
(Lack of foresight & impatience)

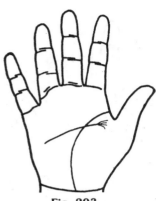

Fig. 203
A bunch like formation of the Head line at the start on the Mount of Mars
(Lack of confidence)

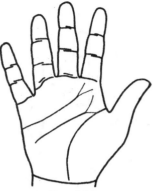

Fig. 204
Line of Head forked at the start, one prong of which goes to the Life line, another to Heart line but not touching the Heart line, and the Heart line also forked
(Good fortune)

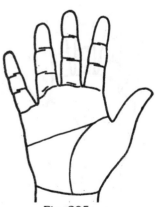

Fig. 205
Extremely long and straight Head line, like a bar
(Extraordinary intellectual powers)

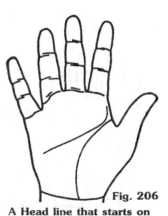

Fig. 206
A Head line that starts on Jupiter then descends to Life line and then goes straight across the hand
(Energy, daring & determination)

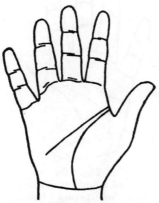

Fig. 207
A straight Head line but slanting
(Cleverness)

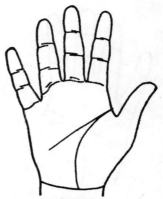

Fig. 208
Head line running close to Life line for sometime
(Brain fever)

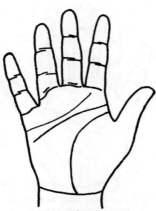

Fig. 209
Head line running close to Heart line
(Asthma, a bigot)

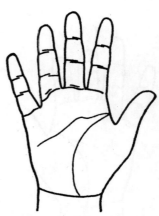

Fig. 210
Head line rising towards the line of Heart under the Mount of Saturn
(Insanity)

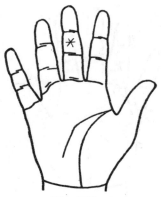

Fig. 211
Head line sloping abruptly to the Mount of Moon with a star on the second phalange of Saturn finger
(Insanity)

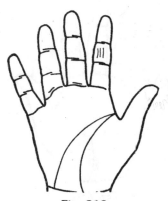

Fig. 212
Head line sweeping down to the wrist with lines on the 2nd phalange of Jupiter finger
(Occultism & Superstition)

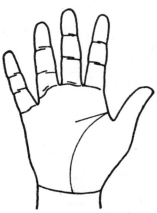

Fig. 213
A short and straight line of Head
(Practical and scientific mind)

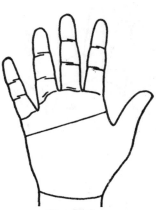

Fig. 214
One straight line as a combination of Head and Heart lines
(Miserly & avaricious disposition)

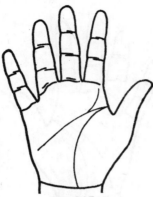

Fig. 215
Rising branch from Head line going to Mount of Jupiter
(Realisation of ambition)

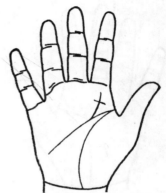

Fig. 216
Rising branch from Head line going to Mount of Jupiter but cut by a bar
(Failure in ambition)

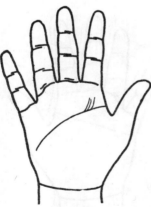

Fig. 217
Three branches from Head line going to the Mount of Jupiter
(Success and riches)

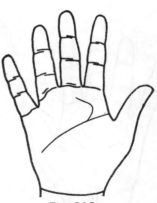

Fig. 218
Rising branch from Head line first going to Jupiter and then to Mount of Saturn
(Vanity & philosophy)

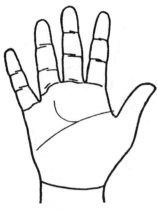

Fig. 219
Rising branch from Head line going to the Mount of Sun
(Success in talents)

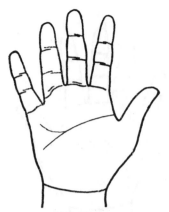

Fig. 220
Rising branch from Head line going to the Mount of Mercury
(Business prosperity)

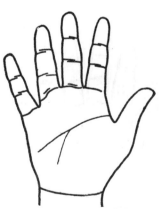

Fig. 221
Rising branch from Head line going to the Mount of Moon
(Love for occultism)

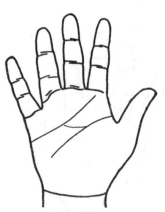

Fig. 222
Rising branch from Head line going to the Line of Heart
(Affection for someone)

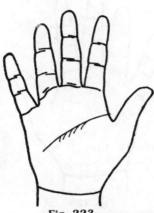

Fig. 223
Falling Branches from Head line
(Anxiety & worry)

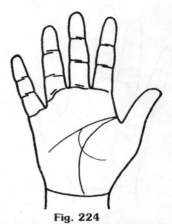

Fig. 224
Falling branch from Head line going to the Mount of Venus
(Forceful love affair)

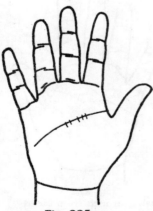

Fig. 225
Bars in the Head line
(Brain disorder, worries)

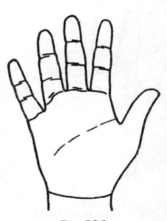

Fig. 226
Breaks in the Head line
(Wound, brain troubles)

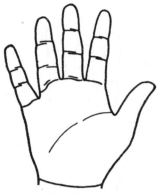

Fig. 227
Head line with a break under the Mount of Saturn, and going to the Mount of Moon
(Insanity)

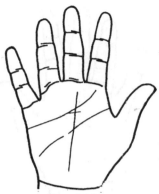

Fig. 228
A break in the Head line and a branch from Heart line cutting the line of Fate
(Widowhood)

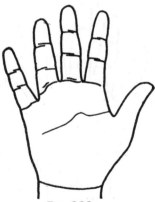

Fig. 229
Head line deflecting towards the Mount of Saturn
(Philosophy, mysticism, melancholia)

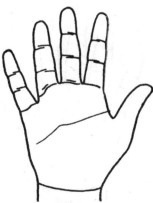

Fig. 230
Head line deflecting towards the Mount of Sun
(Literary activities, enthusiasm)

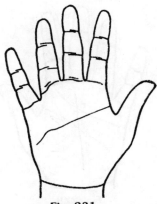

**Fig. 231
Head line deflecting towards
the Mount of Mercury**
*(Business activity, shrewdness,
determination)*

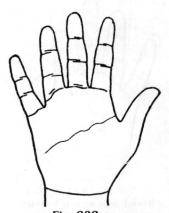

**Fig. 232
Wavy Head line**
(Inconsistency in thought)

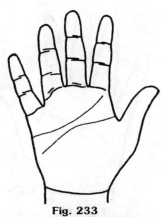

**Fig. 233
Head line deflecting towards
the Heart line**
*(More emotional and
sentimental)*

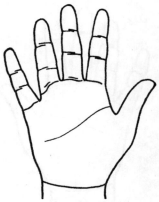

**Fig. 234
Head line deflecting
downwards**
(Mysticism)

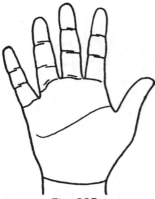

Fig. 235
Head line turning up at its end on the upper Mount of Mars
(Egoism, love of money)

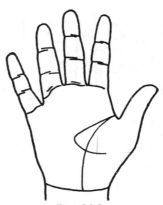

Fig. 236
Head line turning back towards the Mount of Venus
(Cowardice)

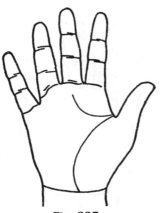

Fig. 237
Head line ending on the Mount of Saturn
(Wound to head and death)

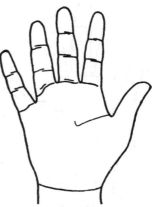

Fig. 238
Head line turns up only towards the Mount of Saturn
(Death by mental paralysis)

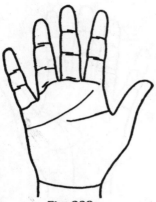

Fig. 239
Head line ending on the Mount of Uranus
(Interest in machinery)

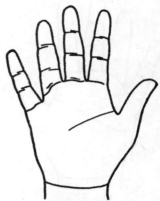

Fig. 240
Head line ending before reaching the Mount of Sun
(Love for art & literature)

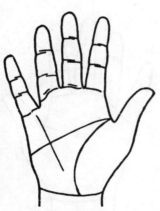

Fig. 241
Head line terminating on the percussion with a good line of Mercury
(Strong memory)

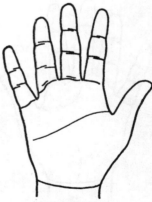

Fig. 242
Head line terminating on the upper Mount of Mars
(Scepticism)

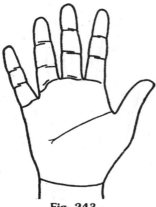

Fig. 243
Head line ending in a small fork
(Versatility)

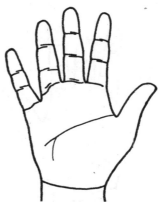

Fig. 244
One prong of the Fork of Head line goes deep to the Mount of Moon
(Hypocrisy & trickery)

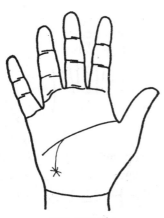

Fig. 245
The prong on the Mount of Moon ends in a star
(Insanity)

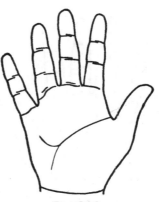

Fig. 246
One fork of the Head line goes to the Mount of Mercury and the other to the Mount of Moon
(Power to hypnotise)

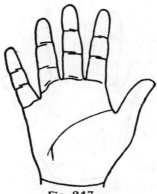

Fig. 247
Head line ending in a fork with both the prongs sloping low down on the Mount of Moon
(Romance)

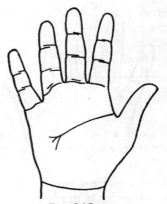

Fig. 248
Head line ending in three prongs
(Mental harmony & Power)

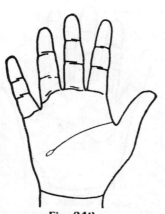

Fig. 249
Head line ending in an island
(Loss of memory)

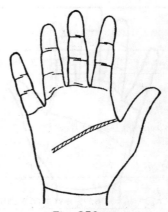

Fig. 250
A broad and shallow Head line
(Lack of courage and force)

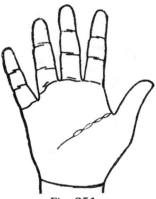

**Fig. 251
Chained line of Head**
(Lack of concentration)

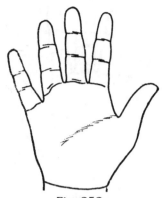

**Fig. 252
Ladder like formation of the
Head line**
(Fickle minded & headaches)

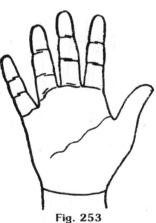

**Fig. 253
Wavy line of Head**
(Lack of mental strength)

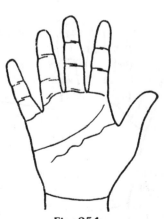

**Fig. 254
Wavy Head line with narrow
Quadrangle**
(A swindler or thief)

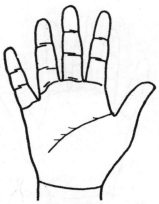

**Fig. 255
Rising splits in the line of Head**
(Aspiration to rise)

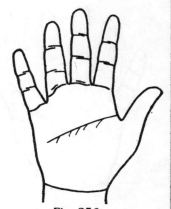

**Fig. 256
Falling splits**
(Sorrow and disappointment)

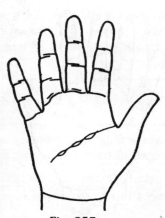

**Fig. 257
Islands in the Head line**
(Brain fever, spirit medium)

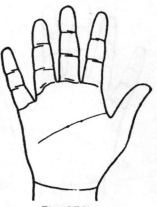

**Fig. 258
Dots in the Head line**
(Brain disorder)

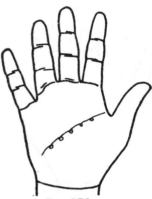

Fig. 259
Knotted Head line
(Tendency to murder)

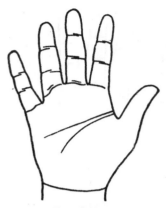

Fig. 260
Double line of Head
(Dual personality, will & determination)

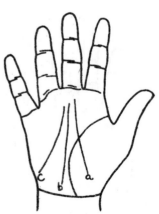

Fig. 261
Three starting positions for the line of Fate
(from inside the Lifeline, centre of the palm, Mount of Moon)

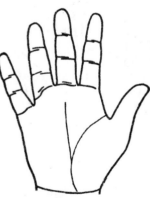

Fig. 262
Fate line starting from Life line
(Success)

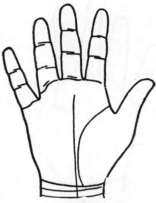

Fig. 263
Fate line starting from the third rascette
(Sorrow & grief)

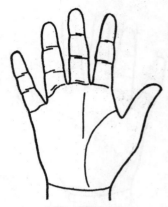

Fig. 264
Fate line starting from the Plain of Mars
(Intelligence, shrewd planning)

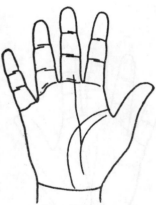

Fig. 265
Fate line starting from the line of Mars and ending into the third phalange of the Saturn finger
(Troubles)

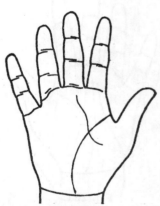

Fig. 266
Crooked line of Fate from Mount of Mars, terminating in the Mount of Saturn
(Imprisonment)

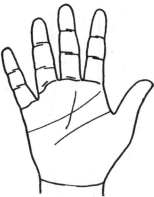

Fig. 267
Fate line starting from the Quadrangle
(Imprisonment or difficulties)

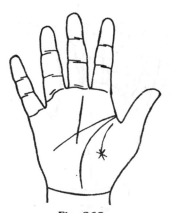

Fig. 268
Fate line starting within the Triangle a parental line ending in a star
(Death of parent prevents good start)

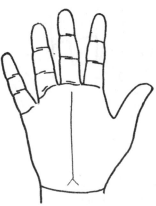

Fig. 269
Fate line starting from a fork
(Adoption)

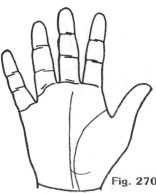

Fig. 270
One prong of Fate line going to the centre of the hand and the other to the Mount of Venus
(Fatal influence of the opposite sex)

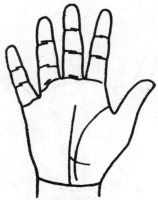

Fig. 271
One prong of the Saturn line going to the Mount of Neptune and the other to the Mount of Venus
(Loss of married partner)

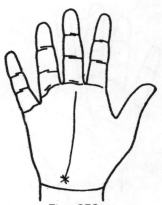

Fig. 272
Fate line starting from a star
(Troubles to parents)

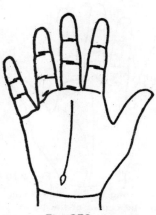

Fig. 273
Fate line starting from an island
(Mystery of birth)

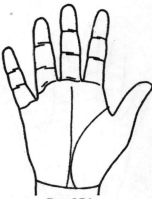

Fig. 274
Fate line running close to Life line for sometime and then going to Mount of Saturn
(Shirking of family responsibilities)

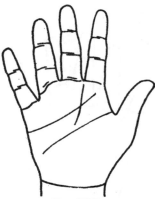

Fig. 275
Fate line starting from the Mount of Uranus and going in between the Jupiter and Saturn fingers
(Wound in lower part of abdomen)

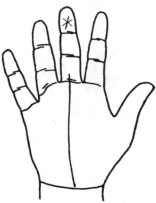

Fig. 276
Deep and red Fate line cutting the third phalange of the Saturn finger, with a star on the first phalange of Saturn finger
(Dishonourable death or imprisonment)

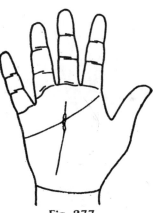

Fig. 277
Chained line of Fate where it crosses the Heart line
(Troubles in love)

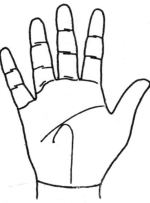

Fig. 278
Fate line turning back in a semi-circular way in the hollow and towards the Mount of Moon
(Imprisonment)

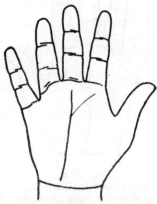

Fig. 279
Rising branch of Fate line going to the Mount of Jupiter
(Creative freedom in art)

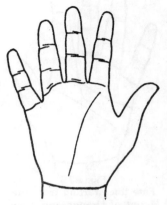

Fig. 280
Fate line ending on the Mount of Jupiter
(Brilliant union)

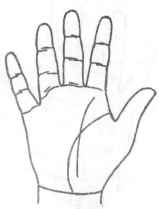

Fig. 281
Fate line starting from the Mount of Venus and ending on the Mount of Jupiter

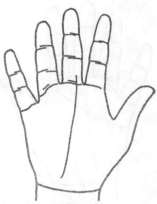

Fig. 282
Fate line pushing into the finger of Saturn
(Unfortunate happenings)

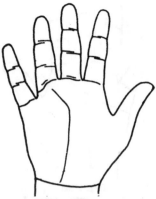

Fig. 283
Fate line ending on the
Mount of Sun
(Celebrity in arts)

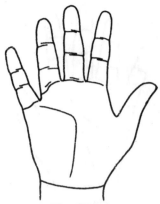

Fig. 284
Fate line ending on the
Mount of Mercury
(Financial prosperity)

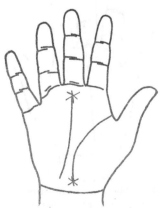

Fig. 285
Fate line and Life line both
ending in star on both the
hands
(Paralysis)

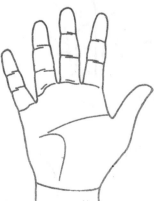

Fig. 286
Fate line ending on the
Upper Mars
(Love of conquest)

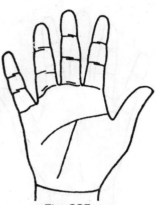

Fig. 287
Fate line ending on Head line
(Loss of career)

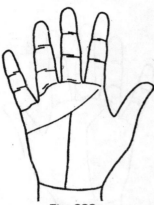

Fig. 288
Fate line starting from 1st Rascette and ending on Heart line
(Troubles in love)

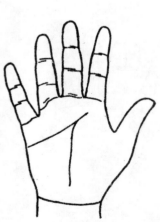

Fig. 289
Fate line merging into the line of Heart
(Brilliant marriage)

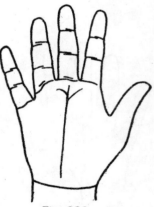

Fig. 290
Fate line ending in three forks one going to the Mount of Jupiter, the other to the Mount of Saturn and the third one to the Mount of Sun
(Wealth, fame & comforts)

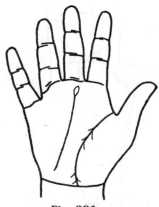

Fig. 291
Fate line ending in an island with falling branches in the Life line
(Unhappy ending of life)

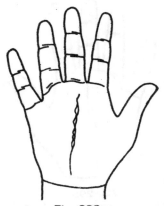

Fig. 292
Chained line of Fate
(Misfortune, hard career)

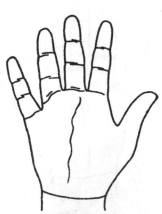

Fig. 293
Wavy line of Fate
(Chequered career, Quarrelsomeness)

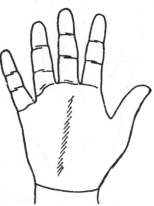

Fig. 294
Ladder like formation of Fate line
(Monetary losses)

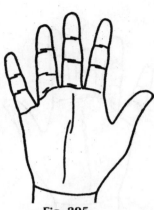

Fig. 295
Overlapping break in Fate line
(Difficulties overcome)

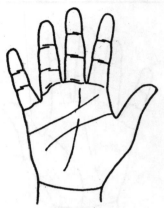

Fig. 296
Fate line broken in the Quadrangle and again starting from the line of Heart
(Fortune due to opposite sex, physical & moral strain)

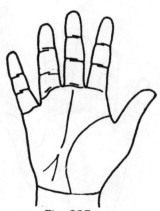

Fig. 297
Fate line starting from a fork, one prong from Mount of Moon, and the line broken at the fork
(Danger from drowning)

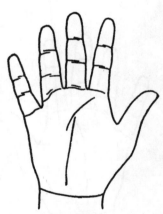

Fig. 298
Overlapping line on the Break in Fate line ending on Mount of Jupiter
(Second marriage)

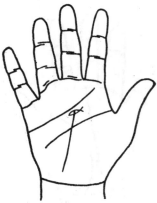

Fig. 299
Island ending in a fork
across the line of Fate and
between the lines of Head &
Heart
(Divorce)

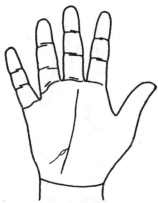

Fig. 300
Island on the Influence line
from Mount of Moon to the
line of Fate
(Misfortune due to union)

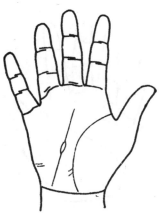

Fig. 301
An island on the Fate line
with many short Travel lines
(Interest in two countries)

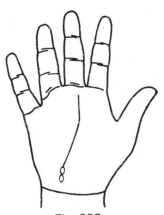

Fig. 302
Fate line starting from two
islands (Figure of eight)
(Gift of second sight)

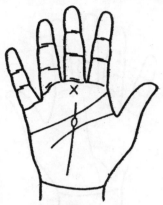

Fig. 303
An island on the Fate line on the Mount of Uranus, with a cross on the Mount of Saturn
(Imprisonment)

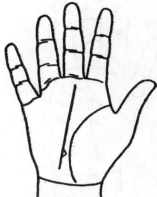

Fig. 304
A Triangle in between the Fate line and the Life line and touching the Fate line
(Military success)

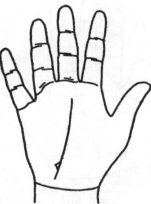

Fig. 305
A Triangle on the Fate line
(Monotonous life)

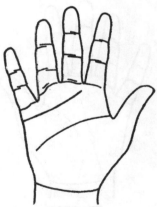

Fig. 306
Heart line placed very high on the hand
(Violent passions & Jealousy)

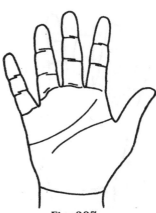

Fig. 307
Heart line placed very low on the hand
(Cold & selfish nature)

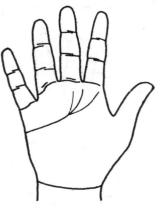

Fig. 308
Heart line starting from all the three positions, viz., Mount of Jupiter, Between Jupiter and Saturn fingers, and from the Mount of Saturn
(Sentiment, commonsense & passion)

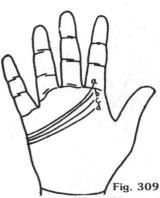

Fig. 309
Heart line starting from
a) 3rd phalange of Jupiter finger. b) base of Jupiter finger. c) middle of Jupiter Mount. d) base of Jupiter Mount

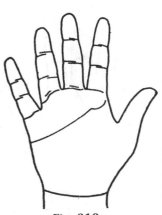

Fig. 310
Heart line encircling the Mount of Jupiter
(Ideal love, occultism, Jealousy)

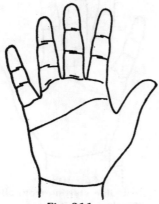

Fig. 311
Heart line starting with a downward curve on the Mount of Jupiter
(Disappointment in love)

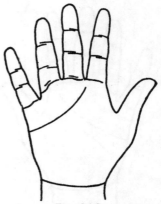

Fig. 312
Heart line starting between Jupiter and Saturn Mounts
(Practical love)

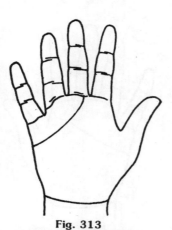

Fig. 313
Heart line starting from finger of Saturn
(Passion & selfishness)

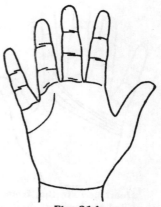

Fig. 314
Heart line starting from the Mount of Sun
(Intense love)

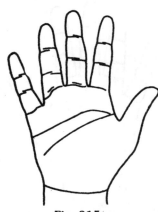

Fig. 315
Heart line starting from the line of Head
(Monetary loss)

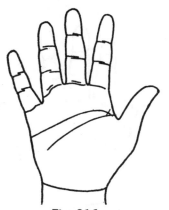

Fig. 316
Small line crossing the Heart line at the time, the Heart line touches the Head line
(Miserable marriage)

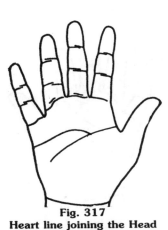

Fig. 317
Heart line joining the Head line under the Mount of Saturn
(Disaster due to passions, Fatal events)

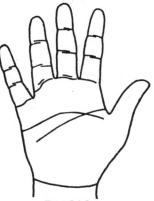

Fig. 318
Heart line starting from the positive Mount of Mars
(Quarrelsome & irritable nature)

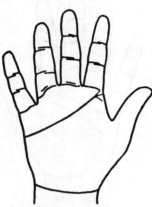

Fig. 319
A fork with three prongs at the edge of the Mount of Jupiter
(Good fortune, happy love)

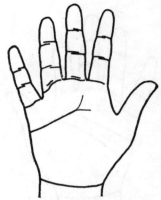

Fig. 320
Fork at the start in Heart line, one prong going to the Mount of Saturn and other to the Head line
(Self deception)

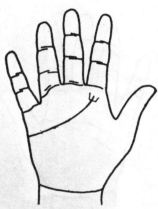

Fig. 321
Trident like formation of the Heart line, on the Mount of Jupiter
(Power of control on others)

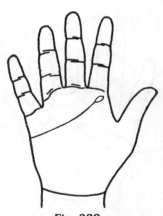

Fig. 322
Heart line starting from an island under the Mount of Jupiter
(Throat and lung troubles)

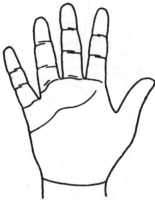

Fig. 323
Heart line rising to Mount of Sun in its course
(Apollonian friends)

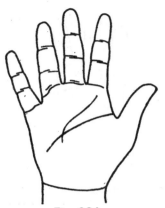

Fig. 324
Heart line cutting the Head line
(Brain fever or death)

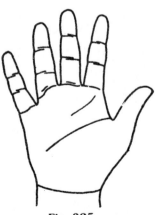

Fig. 325
A short Heart line
(Brutal sexual tendency)

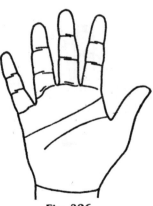

Fig. 326
Heart line crossing the entire hand
(Unhappiness & tyranny in love)

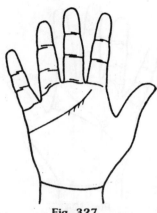

Fig. 327
Falling lines from the Heart line
(Love sorrows)

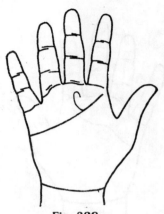

Fig. 328
Rising branch from the Heart line, going to Saturn and then turning back
(Misplaced affection)

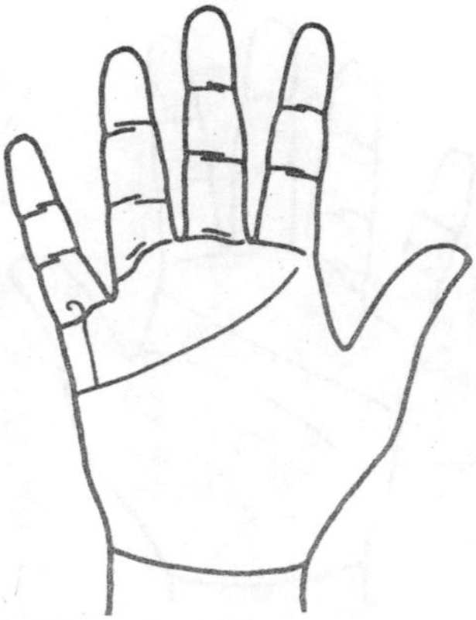

Fig. 329
A straight branch from the Heart line on the finger of Mercury ending in a hook
(Accident to the leg)

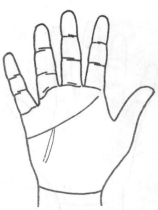

Fig. 330
Two perpendicular lines from the Heart line to the Mount of Moon
(Nervous tension)

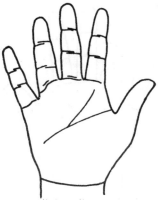

Fig. 331
Heart line ending in Head line
(More of logic & reasoning than emotions)

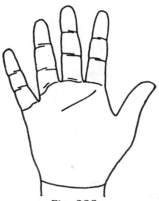

Fig. 332
Heart line ending under Sun
(Attraction towards beauty & arts)

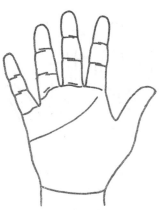

Fig. 333
Heart line ending on upper Mars
(Secretive disposition)

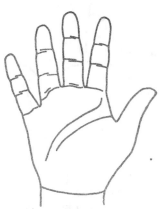

Fig. 334
Heart line ending on Mount of Moon
(Jealousy)

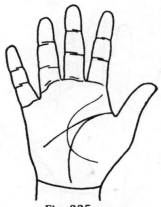

**Fig. 335
Heart line ending on Mount of Venus**
(Danger to head or life)

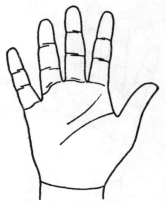

**Fig. 336
Heart line ending in the plain of Mars**
(Irritable nature)

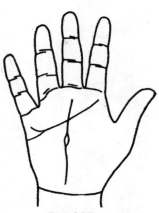

**Fig. 337
Heart line ending in a fork — one prong goes to the Mount of Mercury, with an island in Fate line**
(Divorce)

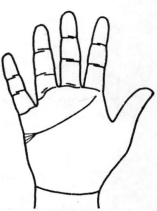

**Fig. 338
Heart line ending in a Tassel**
(Many love affairs)

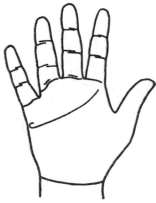

Fig. 339
Heart line ending in a hook on Mercury
(Danger from elephant)

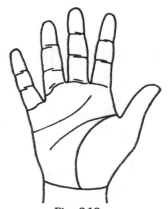

Fig. 340
Narrow and thin line of Heart
(Cowardly & timid disposition)

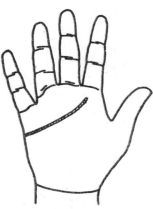

Fig. 341
Broad and shallow Heart line
(A fickle mind)

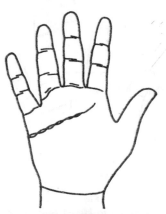

Fig. 342
Chained line of Heart
(A flirt)

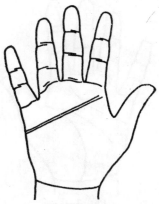

Fig. 343
Rail like line of Heart
(Intense love for wife)

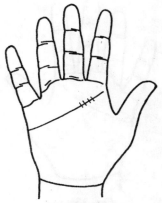

Fig. 344
Cross Bars in Heart line
(Illness or worries)

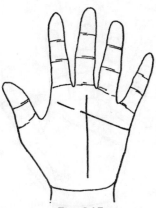

Fig. 345
A break in Heart line on the left side on left hand
(Danger from drowning)

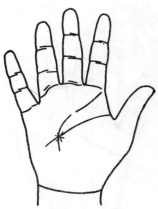

Fig. 346
Broken end of Heart line, cutting the Head line, and a star on the Head line
(Explosion of head)

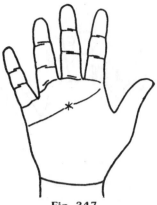

Fig. 347
A star in the break on the
Heart line
(Heart trouble)

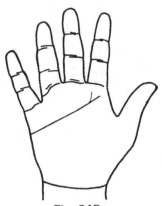

Fig. 348
A rising split on Heart line,
under the Jupiter Mount
(Love guided by ambition)

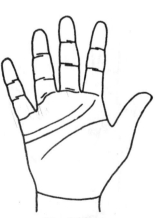

Fig. 349
Double line of Heart
(Sorrow in love)

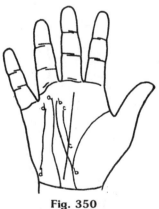

Fig. 350
Line of Sun starting
a) From Rascette
b) From Life line
c) From Fate line
d) From Mount of Moon

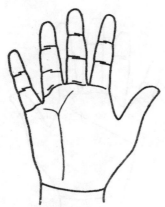

Fig. 351
Sun Line:- One branch goes to Saturn, another to the Mercury Mount
(Wealth & renown)

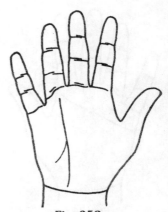

Fig. 352
A branch from Sun line to Moon
(Power of imagination)

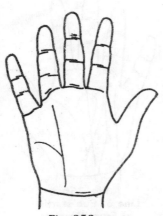

Fig. 353
A branch from Sun line to Upper Mars
(Confidence & self-reliance)

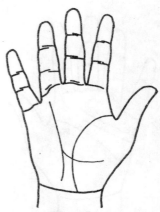

Fig. 354
A branch from Sun line to Venus Mount
(Great love of music)

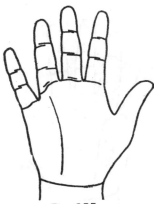

Fig. 355
A Sun line, deep at the start and fading away at the end
(Diminishing wealth)

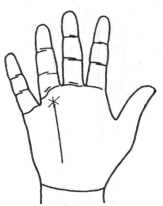

Fig. 356
Sun line ending in a star
(Brilliant success)

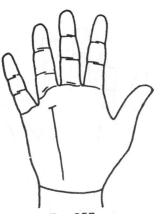

Fig. 357
Sun line ending in a deep bar
(Obstacles in career)

Fig. 358
Sun line ending in three forks — two forks curving in-side
(Opportunity lost & failure)

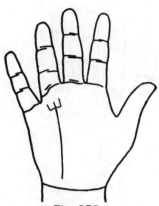

Fig. 359
Sun line ending in a Trident
(Celebrity and wealth)

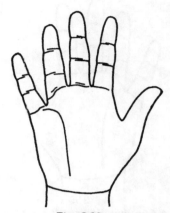

Fig. 360
Sun line ending on Mount of Mercury
(Success in ambition)

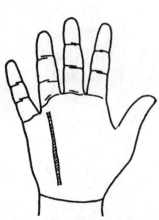

Fig. 361
Broad and shallow line of Sun
(Lack of concentration)

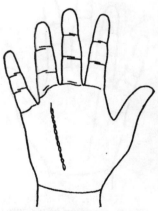

Fig. 362
Chained line of Sun
(Poor success)

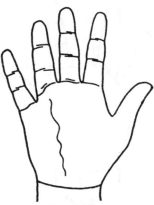

Fig. 363
Wavy line of Sun
(Changing disposition)

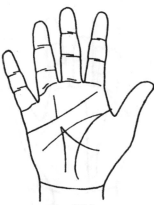

Fig. 364
Sun line broken in the quadrangle, with an influence line from Mount of Venus
(Misfortune)

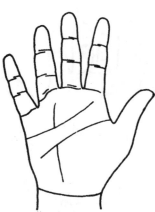

Fig. 365
Sun line broken at the Head line and continues only after the Heart line
(Revival of success)

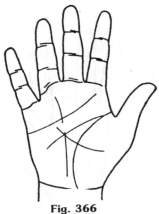

Fig. 366
Sun line broken on the Mount of Uranus, and an influence line from Venus cuts the break
(Series of troubles)

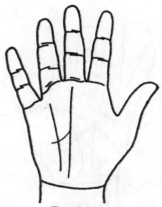

Fig. 367
Line from Fate line, cutting the Sun line
(Failure in partnership)

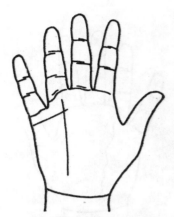

Fig. 368
Sun Line cut by the line of Marriage
(Loss of position due to marriage)

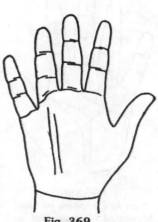

Fig. 369
Double line of Sun
(Unexpected luck and windfall)

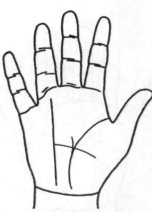

Fig. 370
Influence line from Venus, cutting an upward branch in Life line and touching the line of Sun
(Law suits won)

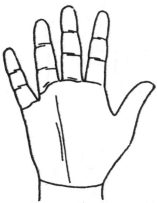

Fig. 371
Influence line running
parallel to Sun Line
(Legacies)

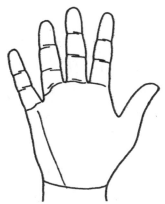

Fig. 372
Mercury line starting from
Rascettes
(Long life)

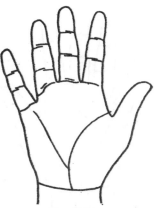

Fig. 373
Mercury line touching the
Life line
(Death)

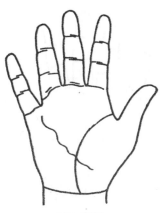

Fig. 374
Wavy Mercury line, starting
from the Mount of Venus
(Immorality)

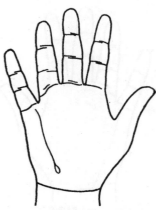

Fig. 375
Mercury line starting from an island
(Somnambulism)

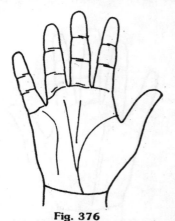

Fig. 376
Mercury line first pointing towards the Mount of Sun and then turning to Mount of Mercury
(Good earning but equal spending)

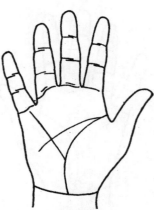

Fig. 377
Mercury line making a triangle with Life line and Head line
(Occultism)

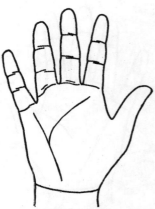

Fig. 378
Branch from Mercury line going to Jupiter Mount
(Success in business)

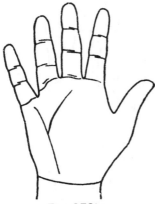

Fig. 379
Branch from Mercury line
going to the Saturn Mount
(Wisdom)

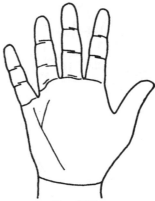

Fig. 380
Branch from Mercury line
going to Mount of Sun
(Shrewdness & success)

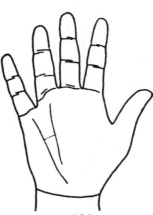

Fig. 381
A line connecting the line of
Sun and the line of Mercury
(Wealth)

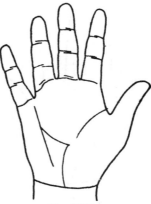

Fig. 382
A branch from Mercury line
touching a break in the Life
line
(Danger of death)

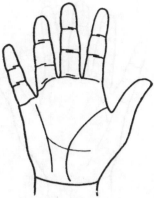

Fig. 383
A branch from Mercury line going to the Mount of Venus
(Warning against theft & deceipt)

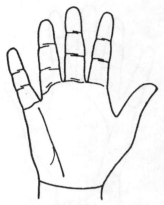

Fig. 384
Branch from Mercury line to Mount of Moon
(Satisfaction in life)

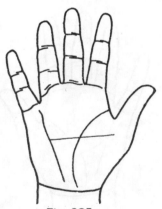

Fig. 385
Line from positive Mars, touching line of Mercury under Mount of Sun
(Purchase of landed property)

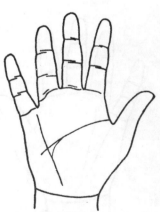

Fig. 386
Branch from Mercury line, merging in Head line
(Succession)

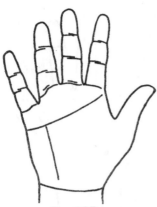

Fig. 387
Mercury line ending on
Heart line
(Heart disease)

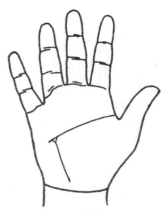

Fig. 388
Mercury line ending in a
fork on Head line
(Love of Honour)

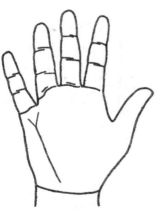

Fig. 389
Mercury line ending in a
fork
(Bad health in old age)

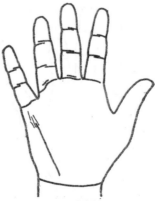

Fig. 390
Mercury line ending by
small lines
(Poverty in old age)

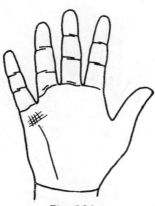

Fig. 391
Mercury line ending in a Grill
(Failure due to poor health)

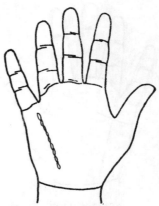

Fig. 392
Chained line of Mercury
(Poor success in business)

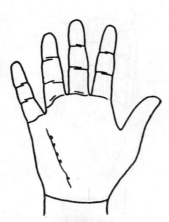

Fig. 393
Twisted line of Mercury
(A thief or a cheat)

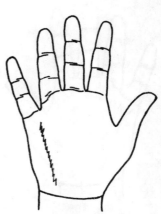

Fig. 394
Ladderlike line of Mercury
(Severe liver trouble)

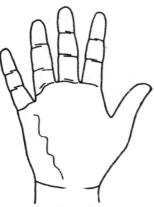

Fig. 395
Wavy line of Mercury
(Billiousness)

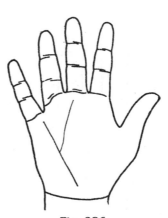

Fig. 396
Line from Saturn Mount touching the line of Mercury
(Luck in race or lottery)

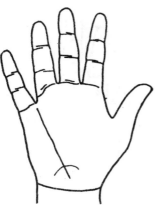

Fig. 397
Line of Mercury cut by via Lasciva
(Liver troubles)

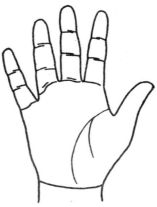

Fig. 398
Line of Mars starting from Life line
(Love affair)

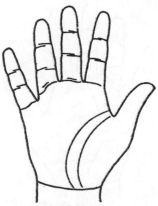

Fig. 399
Line of Mars running full
length to the Life line
(Good health)

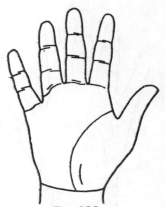

Fig. 400
Line of Mars seen only at
the end of Life line
(Tendency to murder)

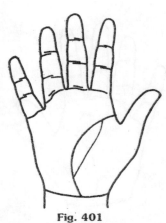

Fig. 401
Line of Mars touching Life
line, at the beginning and
also at the end
(Husband living in the house of wife)

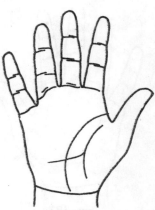

Fig. 402
Branch from Line of Mars
to Moon
(Indulgence in wine & women)

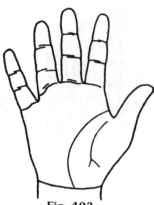

Fig. 403
Line of Mars ending in a fork
(Tendency to murder)

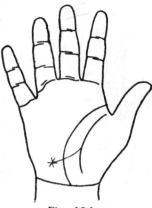

Fig. 404
One of the forks of Line of Mars, ending in a star on Mount of Moon
(Alcoholic insanity)

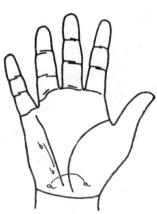

Fig. 405
Two positions of Via Lasciva

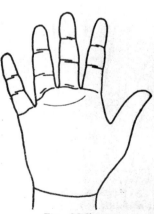

Fig. 406
Girdle of Venus
(Passionate nature)

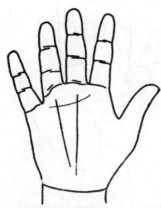

Fig. 407
Girdle of Venus, crossing
lines of Fate & Sun
(Sensual pleasures bar success)

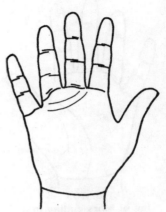

Fig. 408
Double Girdle of Venus
(Lust and intemperance)

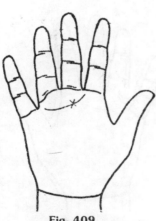

Fig. 409
Cross on Girdle of Venus
under the Mount of Saturn
(Suicide by poison)

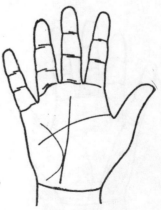

Fig. 410
Line of Intuition making a
triangle with the lines of
Head and Fate
(Occultism)

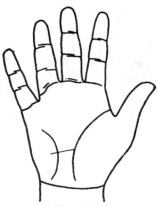

Fig. 411
Line of Influence, from Life line cutting the line of Intuition
(Opposition to the study of occultism)

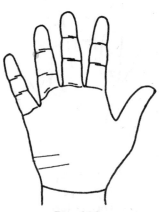

Fig. 413
Travel lines on the Mount of Moon

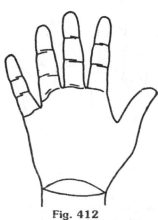

Fig. 412
First Bracelette, curving inside the Palm
(Difficulties in child bearing)

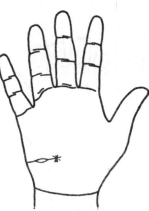

Fig. 414
An island and a star on the Travel line
(Danger from water)

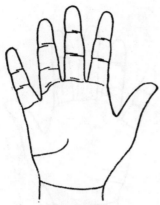

Fig. 415
Line of Voyage turning up towards Mounts
(Advantage through voyage)

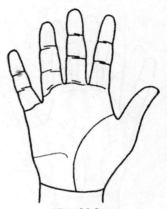

Fig. 416
Line of Voyage turning down towards Life line
(Unsuccessful Journey)

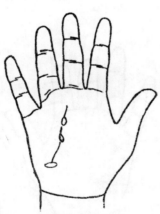

Fig. 417
An island on Mount of Moon joined by an islanded line from Mount of Saturn
(Danger from water)

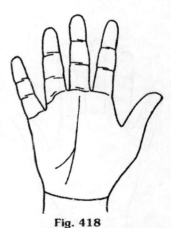

Fig. 418
A line of influence from the Mount of Moon, touching the Line of Fate
(Influence of opposite sex)

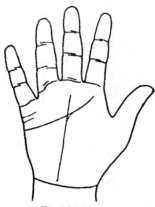

Fig. 419
Two lines of Marriage and a small line from Fate line joining the Heart line on the side of Jupiter
(Second marriage)

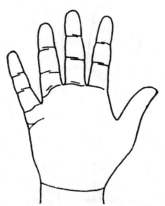

Fig. 420
Marriage line starting with a fork
(Delay in marriage)

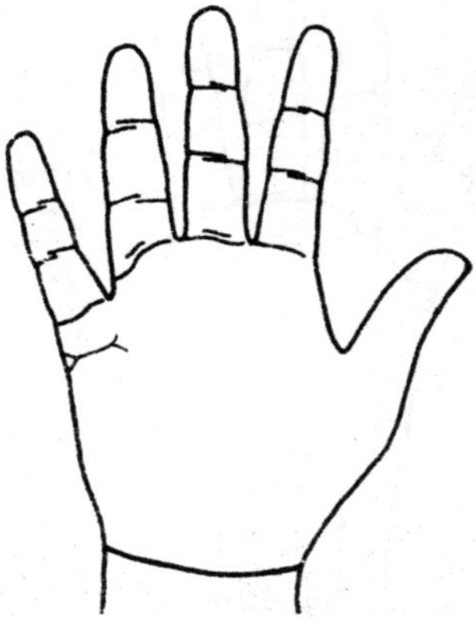

Fig. 421
Forks at both ends of Marriage line
(Separation due to travels)

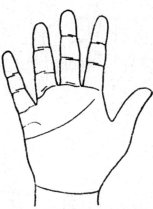

Fig. 422
Marriage line pointing at Heart line
(Quarrels in married life)

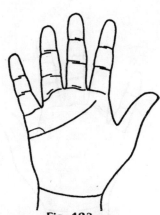

Fig. 423
Marriage line curving down
and touching the Heart line
(Widowhood)

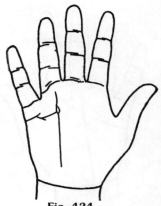

Fig. 424
Marriage line ending in a
fork. A line from the fork
ends in an island on Sun
line
(Scandal & separation)

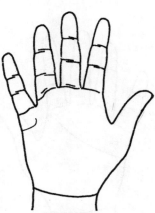

Fig. 425
Marriage line curving
upwards
(No marriage)

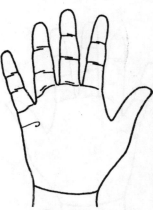

Fig. 426
Marriage line ending in a
hook
(Loss of affection)

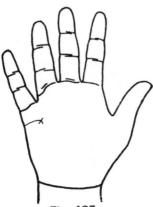

Fig. 427
A bar line cutting a dropping line of Marriage
(Sudden death of partner)

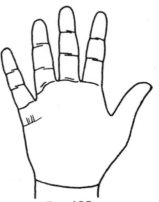

Fig. 428
Lines of children

INDEX OF SIGNS ON THE HAND

CROSS:

1. A cross or line on the second phalange of Jupiter finger shows rich friends.
2. A cross on the Mount of Jupiter means happy marriage.
3. A clear cross on the Mount of Jupiter denotes:
   (a) Love for one person only.
   (b) Wealthy marriage.
   (c) Happy marriage.
4. A cross on the Mount of Saturn indicates:
   (a) Childlessness.
   (b) Murder or assassination.
   (c) Misuse of occult power.
   (d) Ill-health.
   (e) Sterility.
5. A cross on the first phalange of Apollo finger on a woman's hand shows chastity.
6. A cross on the Mount of Apollo indicates:
   (a) Financial troubles.
   (b) Reverse of fortune.
7. A cross on the first phalange of Mercury finger means that the person may remain unmarried.
8. A cross on the Mount of Mercury denotes:
   (a) Financial troubles.
   (b) Wound on legs.
   (c) A liar.
   (d) Syphilis.
9. A cross on the upper Mount of Mars denotes stealing.
10. A cross on the lower Mount of Mars means suicidal tendency.
11. A cross on the plain of Mars indicates death by execution.
12. A cross on the Mount of Venus touching the line of Life indicates troubles from relatives.
13. A large cross on the Mount of Venus denotes love for one person only.
14. A cross cutting the middle Mount of Moon means suffering from rheumatism.

15 A cross on the lower third of the Mount of Moon speaks of bladder or kidney troubles.
16 A cross in the Quadrangle under the Mount of Saturn is an indication of:
   (a) Fortunate and lucky life.
   (b) Priesthood.
   (c) Occultism.
   (d) Clairvoyance.
17 A cross on the line of Life tells of law suits.
18 A cross on the break in the line of Fate indicates a most critical change in the person's life.
19 A cross at the centre of the Fate line means disastrous change.
20 A cross on the Heart line at the intersection of the Fate line shows pecuniary troubles due to love matters.

STAR

1 A star on the Mount of Jupiter denotes:
   (a) Wealthy marriage.
   (b) Public honours.
   (c) Accident from fire.
2 A star at the edge of the Jupiter Mount and touching the line of Life shows loss of mother.
3 A star at the edge of the Jupiter Mount but not touching the Life line tells of illegitimate birth.
4 A star on the Mount of Saturn on both the hands means death on the scaffold.
5 A star between the Mounts of Saturn and Apollo means danger from electricity or snake-bite.
6 A star on the Mount of Mercury shows:
   (a) Stealing.
   (b) Forgery.
   (c) Loss by theft or treachery.
   (d) Embezzler or highway robber.
7 A star on the upper Mount of Mars denotes:
   (a) Military honour.
   (b) Death in war.
8 A star in the centre or at the base of the Mount of Venus means

success in love.
9. A star on the lower Mount of Moon indicates:
   (a) Mysterious life.
   (b) Alcoholic insanity.
   (c) Hysteria.
10. A star on the line of Mercury denotes unexpected luck. It also means not more than one child.

VERTICAL LINES

1. Four vertical lines on the second and third phalanges of Jupiter finger is a sign of happy and virtuous life.
2. A vertical line on the Mount of Saturn indicates happy old age.
3. Two vertical lines on the Mount of Saturn, one on the side of Apollo and the other on the side of Jupiter indicates:
   (a) Happy maternity.
   (b) Male offspring.
4. Two clear-cut lines on the Mercury finger denote a nursing profession.
5. Short vertical lines near the nail of the thumb is an indication of legacy.
6. Vertical lines on the second joint of the thumb mean brothers.

HORIZONTAL LINES

1. A cross line on the third joint of Jupiter finger indicates a tendency towards acquisition of the property of others.
2. Cross lines on the Mount of Moon indicate voyage.
3. Wavy cross lines on the first phalange of all fingers show danger from drowning.

CIRCLE

1. A circle on the Mount of Jupiter means remembrance of previous birth.
2. A circle on the Mount of Mercury indicates danger from water and also from poisoning.
3. One circle on the Life line shows susceptibility to blindness of one eye.

4 Two circles on the Life lihe show total blindness.
5 A circle on the Mercury line denotes minor misfortunes during hunting or driving.

TRIANGLE

1 A triangle on the Mount of Jupiter denotes a diplomat.
2 A triangle on the Mount of Saturn speaks of occultism.
3 A triangle on the Mount of Sun indicates success in the arts.
4 A triangle on the Mount of Moon gives intuition.
5 A triangle on the Life line means that the person will support the families of relatives and friends.
6 A triangle on the Fate line indicates a monotonous life.
7 A triangle attached to the line of Heart in the Quadrangle denotes periods of income and improvement in financial position.
8 A triangle with a cross in it in first bracelette speaks of a large fortune through inheritance

ISLAND OR YAVA

1 An island or yava on the second joint of Saturn finger brings wealth through adoption, lottery or inheritance.
2 An island under the Mount of Saturn indicates deafness.
3 An island in the Head line under the Mount of Saturn is a sign of deafness.
4 An island at the beginning of the Fate line speaks of the mystery of birth.

ALPHABETICAL INDEX

Ability to impart mental peace and solace:
Line of Life ending on the Mount of Neptune and the Mercury line touching the Life line.

Accident:

(a) **From fire:** A star on the outer edge of Jupiter Mount.

(b) **To the head:** A break in the line of Head.

(c) **Accident crippling the person, generally the legs:** A straight branch from the Heart line ending in a hook on the finger of Mercury.

(d) **From motor car:** Rising line from the Life line going upto the Saturn Mount.

Achievement in scientific pursuits:

(a) A rising branch of Head line going between 3rd and 4th fingers.

(b) The Head line terminating between the line of Sun and the Mercury finger.

Acquisition of other's money: A cross line on the third joint of Jupiter finger.

Acquisition of property, land or agriculture: Small triangle on the line of Life.

Ambassador: All the three phalanges of Mercury finger equal in length and the Head line having branches.

Architect: A sloping line of Head with spatulate fingers.

Arrogance:

(a) Excess development of Jupiter Mount.

(b) Wide gap between Head and Life lines.

Art of mimicry: Line of Head reaching upto the line of Heart but not touching it.

Assasination:

(a) A star on the Mount of Saturn at the end of Fate line.

(b) A cross or star on the Mount of Mars.

(c) A large cross in the centre of the big Triangle.

(d) A black spot at the end of broken line of Life.

Asthma:

(a) Narrow Quadrangle with a poor line of Mercury.

(b) Hedge-like formation on the line of life.

Author of scientific books: Sign of Uranus on the Mount of Mercury.

Author of children's stories: Sign of Neptune on the Mount of Mercury.

Banker: A rising branch from the Mercury line to the Mount of Saturn.

Blindness:

(a) Star in the Triangle touching the line of Mercury.

(b) Circle on the line of Life.

Blood poisoning: Presence of double or triple or broken Girdle of Venus.

Brothers:

(a) Vertical lines on the second joint of thumb.

(b) Vertical lines on the Mount of Venus and parallel to the line of Mars.

Businessman:

(a) Long second phalange of Mercury.

(b) Fate line starting from the Mount of Moon.

Career : Career abroad: A straight line of voyage on the Mount of Moon with a break in the Fate line.

   Change of career: A break in the Fate line.

   Loss of career: One prong of Head line going to the Mount of Moon and another touching the line of Heart.

Corporal punishment: Absence of the Mount of Saturn.

Cautious:

(a) Close carriage of the thumb.

(b) Life line closely connected to Head line.

Children:

(a) Fork at the end of the Heart line.

(b) Islands or Yavas on the second phalange of the thumb.

(c) Small lines on the upper Mount of Mars.

(d) Falling lines from the Heart line on the upper Mount of Mars.

(e) Lines on second phalanges of Mercury and Saturn fingers.

(f) Vertical lines on the first phalange of Jupiter or Apollo finger.

(g) Vertical lines on the first phalange of the thumb.

(h) Two vertical lines on either side of the Mount of Saturn.

No Children:

(a) Cross on the Mount of Saturn.

(b) Star at the juncture of crossing of Head and Mercury lines.

(c) Heart line ending branchless.

Twins: Two lines of children rising from the same point.

Clairvoyance: Mercury line forms a small triangle with the lines of Head and Life.

Humbug Clairvoyant:

(a) A poor Mercury line with the presence of Intuition line.

(b) A cross on the line of Intuition with a badly marked Mount of Mercury.

Gift of Clairvoyance: Line of Intuition starting from an island.

Criminal:

(a) Double thumb.

(b) Clubbed thumb.

(c) Black spots on the nail of the thumb.

Criminal jealousy:

(a) Excess of the Mount of Jupiter.

(b) A Saturnian with yellow colour.

(c) Bad Mercurian.

Criminal tendency:

(a) Absence of the Heart line on a bad hand.

(b) Yellow colour of the Heart line.

(c) Head line terminating on the Heart line.

Cruelty:

(a) Narrow Quadrangle with Mars or Mercury strong.

(b) Absence of Heart line with negative Mount of Mars very prominent.

Culprit: Grill on the Mount of Saturn.

Danger from drowning or shipwreck:

(a) A star on the voyage line.

(b) Circle on the Mount of Moon.

(c) A cross on the Mount of Moon.

(d) Wavy cross lines on first phalanges of all fingers.

(e) An island on the line of voyage.

Danger from electricity: Star between the Mounts of Saturn and Apollo.

Danger from fire:
(a) Heart line broken at the right side of the right hand.
(b) A wavy line cutting the Heart line from below.
(c) A star on the outer edge of Jupiter finger.

Danger from high fall:
Two vertical lines in the middle of the Heart line.

Danger through horse riding: Oblique bar across the Heart line on Jupiter Mount.

Deafness:
(a) An island in the centre of the Mount of Saturn.
(b) A black spot on the line of Head with a fork at the start in the Life line.
(c) A black spot on a line from upper Mount of Mars to the Mount of Jupiter.
(d) An island in the line of Head under Saturn Mount.

Desire fulfilled: A Mercury line throwing a branch towards the Mount of Moon.

Desire for power: Jupiter finger equal to Saturn finger.

Devotion to friends: A Martian.

Dexterity: A Mercurian.

Dictatorship and cruelty: Life line starting high on the Mount of Jupiter.

Divorce:
(a) An island ending in a fork across the line of Fate and between the lines of Head and Heart.
(b) A rising branch from Life line cut by a line from the Mount of Mars or Venus.
(c) Cross line from Mount of Mars or Venus cutting the line of Marriage.
(d) Marriage line ending in a fork.

Ear trouble: A Saturnian.

Enemies:
(a) A grill in the Triangle.
(b) Lines from bracelets reaching the Moon Mount.

Engineer:
(a) Spatulate tip to Mercury finger.
(b) Flat Mounts.

(c) Broad palm.

Egoism: Too wide a gap between the lines of Life and Head.

Eye trouble:

(a) An Apollonian.

(b) Circle on the Sun Mount.

(c) A break in Head line under the Sun Mount.

(d) An island in the Heart line under Sun.

(e) A circle in the Heart line under Sun.

Failure at the eleventh moment: Crooked finger of Sun.

Failure in realising ambitions: A rising branch of Head line ending in a bar.

Falsehood: Triangle at the end of Life line.

Financial difficulties: Life line ending in a fork.

> **In old age:** Entire space between the lines of Head and Heart filled with an island.
>
> **Due to law-suits:** Deep lines from the line of Head cutting the Fate line.

Foreign travels: Stay in Foreign Country:

(a) Life line ending deep into the Mount of Moon.

(b) An influence line from the Mount of Moon.

Fortune in old age:

(a) Chained first bracelet.

(b) Straight Fate line starting from the line of Heart.

Gambler:

(a) Finger of Apollo longer than the finger of Saturn.

(b) Large Mount of Moon.

(c) Soft hands.

Tricky gambler: Crooked finger of Apollo which is longer than the Saturn finger.

Genius misdirected: Two parallel wavy lines on either side of the straight and deep line of Sun.

Hypnotic powers:

(a) Upper Mount of Mars leaning towards Moon.

(b) Mount of Mercury leaning towards Upper Mars.

(c) Sign of Saturn on the Mount of Saturn.

Idiots:

(a) High set or powerless thumb.

(b) One of the main lines missing.

Imprisonment:

(a) A square touching the Life line from inside.

(b) Fate line starting from the Quadrangle.

(c) Fate line turning back in a semi-circular way towards the Mount of Moon and ending in the hollow.

(d) An island on the Fate line on the Mount of Uranus and a cross on the Mount of Saturn.

(e) Deep Fate line cutting third phalange of Saturn finger.

Indulgence in wine and women:

(a) Branch from line of Mars going to Mount of Moon.

(b) Line of Via Lasciva ending on the Mount of Moon.

Intuition:

(a) Development of the first phalange of the Jupiter finger.

(b) A Mercurian.

(c) A triangle on the Mount of Moon.

(d) Fate line starting from two islands.

Jack of all trades: Square hand with mixed fingers of different shapes.

Journey:

(a) **Both by land and sea:** A rising branch from bracelet. Via Lasciva starting either from the line of Fate or the line of Mercury and going to the Mount of Moon unbroken and uniformly constituted.

(b) **Fortunate journey:** The line of Via Lasciva extending upto the Mount of Moon and going downward into it.

(c) **Successful and profitable journey:** A cross or an angle or a star on a rising branch from bracelet going to the Mount of Jupiter. Two lines from the bracelet going across the Mount of Moon.

Law suits:

(a) Cross on the Life line.

(b) Cross inside the upper angle of the Triangle.

(c) Two or more forks at the start of the Life line under the Mount of Jupiter.

Law suits due to death: An influence line from a star cutting a short upward branch of the line of Life.

Loss of Law suits: An influence line from a star cutting a branch of the Life line and this line cutting the line of Sun.

Success in law suits: An influence line from an island crossing the upward branch of the Life line and merging into the line of Sun.

Legacy:

(a) Small vertical lines near the nail of the thumb.

(b) Sign of Yava or lotus on the thumb.

(c) Star on the first bracelet.

(d) Cross in the Big Triangle.

Love affairs:

(a) A single vertical line on the Mount of Venus going to the Mount of positive Mars.

(b) **Love affair met with frustration:** Two lines from the Mount of Venus meeting on a star on the Fate line.

(c) **Love affair forced on the individual:** Falling branch from the line of Head going to the Mount of Venus.

(d) **Guilty love affair:** An island on the Fate line with a star on the Jupiter Mount.

(e) **Tragedy in love affair:** (i) Head, Heart and Life lines closely connected. (ii) Wide break in the Heart line.

Marriage (happy):

(a) Cross on the Mount of Jupiter.

(b) Double line of influence on the Mount of Venus.

(c) A sister line to the Fate line.

(d) An influence line from the Mount of Moon merging in the Fate line.

(e) Presence of Girdle of Venus only on one hand.

(f) A deep and well-cut line of Marriage

Marriage (more than one):

(a) Thicker finger of Saturn.

(b) Two marriage lines.

(c) A break in the Fate line and the overlapping line ending on the Mount of Jupiter.

Marriage (late): A Saturnian. Marriage line starting with a fork or an island.

Marriage (absence of):

(a) A cross on the first phalange of the Mercury finger.

(b) An influence line on the Mount of Venus turning away from the Life line.

(c) Marriage line curving upwards.

Occultism:

(a) A rising branch from the Head line going to the Mount of Mo

(b) Heart line encircling the Mount of Jupiter.

(c) Mercury line ending in a fork on the Head line so as to form a triangle with the Head line.

(d) St. Andrews cross in the Quadrangle.

(e) Two or three vertical lines on the middle phalange of Mercury finger.

Quarrelsome:

(a) A cross in the centre of the Big Triangle.

(b) A Martian with stiff hand.

(c) Short but broad nails.

(d) Wide gap between Head and Life lines.

Riches:

(a) Two lines from the first phalange of the thumb going to the line of Life.

(b) Prominent line on the first joint of the thumb.

(c) Many lines on Apollo finger from the root going to the first phalange.

(d) Long and uncrossed line of Sun.

(e) Double line of Life.

Snake bite: A star between the Mounts of Saturn and Sun.

Voyage:

(a) Horizontal line on the middle of Mount of Moon from the side of percussion.

(b) A line from bracelets going to the Mount of Jupiter.

Voyage for business: Voyage line turning up and joining the line of Head.